It's Your Body

It's Your Body

The Young Woman's Guide to Empowered Sexual Health

DENA MOES, RN, CNM

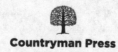

Countryman Press

An Imprint of W. W. Norton & Company
Independent Publishers Since 1923

Page 40: How Well Does Birth Control Work? © 2013–2023, The Regents of the University of California and the Power to Decide. All Rights Reserved.

Page 12: iStock / Daria Kozlova; page 16: iStock / Mary Long; page 21: iStock / Pikovit44; page 22: iStock / Pikovit44; page 26: iStock / Koyuki; page 28: iStock / Daria Kozlova; page 32: iStock / Aleksei Morozov; page 36: iStock / Anna Bova; page 42: iStock / Marina Vishtak; page 53: iStock / RobinOlimb; page 63: iStock / RobinOlimb; page 88: iStock / Inna Miller; page 90: iStock / Kei; page 119: iStock / blueringmedia; page 135: iStock / Anastasia Usenko; page 165: iStock / CARME PARRAMON

For information about permission to reproduce selections from this book, write to Permissions, Countryman Press, 500 Fifth Avenue, New York, NY 10110

For information about special discounts for bulk purchases, please contact W. W. Norton Special Sales at specialsales@wwnorton.com or 800-233-4830

Manufacturing by Lakeside Book Company
Book design by Chris Welch
Production manager: Anna Oler

Countryman Press
www.countrymanpress.com

An imprint of W. W. Norton & Company, Inc.
500 Fifth Avenue, New York, NY 10110
www.wwnorton.com

978-1-68268-889-2

10 9 8 7 6 5 4 3 2 1

This book is dedicated to the freedom and dignity

of everyone's daughters,

in this moment

and all the moments yet to come.

"Like the two wings of a bird, women and men
are of equal value. For without the two in perfect
balance, humanity cannot progress."

—*Amma*

"Each time a woman stands up for herself, without
knowing it possibly, without claiming it,
she stands up for all women."

—*Maya Angelou*

Contents

Introduction

Welcome to *It's Your Body*.

This book is written just for *you*, young women, folks who menstruate, and the people who care about them. It is a guidebook to your body, birth control, safe sex, and what to do if you get pregnant.

This book is titled "It's Your Body" because when it comes to your life, your health, your decisions, it starts there. With your body. Yours. Relationships and romantic partners will come and go throughout your life, but your relationship with yourself is going to last a lifetime.

The transition from child to adult happens in the few short years of adolescence—a whirlwind of life and body changes. A few years ago you were a kid, and now you are suddenly inhabiting a mature body. Interest in romance, intimacy, and sex may arise for you. Sex as a young person can be playful and pleasurable, but it can also have serious adult consequences.

Social media, movies, and the internet send so many confusing messages about female bodies and sex, it's hard to know how best to approach sex in order to have safe and positive experiences. On top of that, your access to reproductive health care options may be limited now because of where you live. On June 24, 2022, the US Supreme Court overturned *Roe v. Wade*, which was the landmark 1973 Supreme Court decision that guaranteed the right to abortion for people in the United States. Until then, abortion had been a guaranteed constitutional right in this country. Since the overturn, the laws regarding access to birth control and abortion are changing around the country, state by state. It is confusing for everybody—young people like you, doctors, health care providers, activists, and policymakers.

No matter where in the world you live, I want you to take an empowered approach to your sex life so you are not derailed by unintended consequences and can live to your full potential. I am going to give you the facts about your period, birth control, and the health issues around sex so you can make your own choices. No matter what is going on with politics or social media, your body is your business. How you take care of it now will affect your entire life.

My purpose here is to give you tools to do that well.

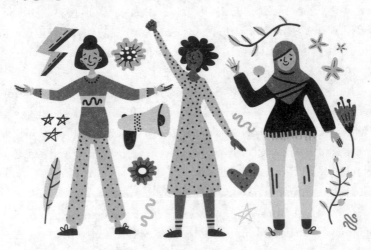

For 22 years I have worked in the state of California, where every person has the right to reproductive health care, regardless of age, without the need for parental notification or consent. Under California law, everyone has the right to birth control, emergency contraception, pregnancy testing, prenatal care, abortion services, and testing and treatment for sexually transmitted infections (STIs) at any age, period. You do not need permission from anyone, including your parents or guardians *or* your partner. It is your right to get these health services confidentially—the clinic or doctor cannot tell anyone why you were there unless you say it's okay. You also can leave school to access these services without getting permission from or telling your parents or guardians. *It's your body.*

This book is written in the same spirit as that California law. I am assuming you, my reader, are at a stage in your life where you are thinking about or engaging in sexual activity. This book is a guide to approaching sex in an informed and healthy way to reduce your risk of an unintended pregnancy, STIs, and sexual assault. And it will provide information on what to do if those things do happen to you.

In this book you will learn about:

* Your menstrual cycle
* Birth control methods: what they are, how well they work, how to use them correctly, side effects, and things to consider when choosing a method
* Emergency contraception
* STIs
* Vaginal infections and vaginal health
* An understanding of female-bodied sexual pleasure
* Consent, boundaries, and sexual assault awareness

* Pregnancy options: continuing the pregnancy, adoption, and abortion
* Surgical and medical abortion, and how to use abortion medications safely
* Resources for accessing all of the services above

My name is Dena, and my pronouns are she/her. I am a registered nurse (RN) and certified nurse-midwife (advanced practice nurse). I have a master's degree in nursing from Yale University, and I am an expert in women's health. My career began in my early 20s, when I became a nurse-midwife because I wanted to be of service to the women of the world.

Midwife means "with woman," and midwives aim to provide health care in which women are listened to, respected, and have agency over their own bodies. Midwives' care focuses on education and empowerment, with the core values of equity, justice, and respect for human dignity.

I trained at Yale and in hospitals in the Bronx, New York, then worked in reproductive health care in California for 22 years. Early in my career, I worked in several different hospitals, and then, for over a decade, I cared for pregnant mothers and delivered hundreds of babies in my own home birth service. For the past six years, I've worked in a free/low-cost feminist health clinic, where I have helped thousands of teens and young people with birth control, STIs, and other reproductive health issues, including unintended pregnancy. At this clinic, I have also provided gender-affirming hormone therapy to transgender people.

I thought about writing this book for a long time because I

share the same information to one person at a time in my clinic, day after day, year in and year out. I have often thought that I should just put this all in a book instead. With the changes happening around the country after the overturn of *Roe v. Wade*, the time to arm young people with knowledge and smart decision-making is *now*.

> "I am not free while any woman is unfree, even when
> her shackles are very different from my own."
> —*Audre Lorde*

The purpose of this book is to help people make informed choices about their sexual health. It is written from a feminist perspective, grounded in the principles of equity and dignity for all people. I believe that girls, women, and people who menstruate have the right to a dignified, fulfilled life with the same opportunities and autonomy as boys and men. And I am well acquainted with the reality that there are social, economic, and political structures in place that favor men and boys over women and girls. Laws that block access to abortion care and contraception perpetuate that inequality because they negatively impact women and girls.

The task of feminism is to make things more equal among people regardless of gender, gender identity, sex, and sexual orientation. I am an intersectional feminist, meaning I am aware that race and racism in America impacts people's lives and opportunities as well. This book is feminist because when girls and women control their fertility, they have increased agency in all aspects of life, such as sports, arts, education, and career.

Other than being feminist, this book has no religious or political affiliation or agenda. I have no vested interest in any contraceptive method, drug, treatment, or clinic.

In places where women don't have access to reproductive health options, they spend most of their lives, from puberty to menopause, having babies and raising children. This can be a wonderful, fulfilling life, but it should be a *choice*. And children should not be forced to have children. The thing is, over the course of your life, you can actually do it all—sports, education, career, travel, and, when you are ready, have children too.

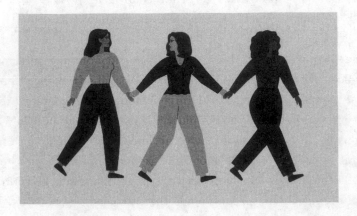

I am going to give you the facts about birth control, sexual health, and abortion so you can make *informed decisions* about your body. Misinformation about these subjects circulates everywhere—on the internet, in schools, and even within families. While it is legit to question the safety of birth control methods and you should know the risks associated with them before using them, it is important to discern between anecdotal stories and facts. Hearsay is what you hear from people who are not health care providers, such as friends, relatives, even your mom, or someone at school. "I heard this happened to a girl on birth control . . ." Rumors often start with the phrase "I heard that . . ."

Facts are proven truths based on data from large studies. Every method of birth control and abortion discussed in this book has been proven safe by exhaustive clinical trials involving hundreds of thousands of people. If you have questions about birth control, it is best to talk to a licensed health care provider, such as the nurse-midwife at a family planning clinic, your doctor, or a telehealth nurse. This book gives you information based on medically researched *facts*. To illustrate facts, I will share examples and stories based on things I have personally seen as a health care provider. Names and other characteristics are all made up to protect everyone's privacy.

It can be tricky to find reliable information about these topics on the internet. Internet searches for information about birth control or abortion often lead searchers to **fake clinics**—websites set up by antiabortion and anticontraception activists to look legitimate but intending to trick you and steer you away from accessing the services that could make your life safer and better. These fake clinics and fake websites are everywhere! The people behind them are very deceptive and determined, and do not have your best interest in mind. It can be very hard to tell what is real medical information and what is false information on the internet. I provide reliable websites for further research at the end of each chapter.

How Should I Use This Book?

Use it any way you want. Really. Flip through it, read about only what interests you. Satisfy your curiosity about different birth control methods. Share it with a friend. Read through it with a parent or trusted relative. Put it on the shelf and keep it in case you need it later. If you have ordered birth control online and are confused about how to use it correctly, look it up here. If you or a friend are pregnant, skip to that section. If someone you know has bought medical abortion pills online, loan them this book because it contains instructions on how to take them correctly and safely. Read about STIs, get a healthy dose of concern, and then go get yourself tested at your student health center or public health department. There is no wrong way to use this book.

A Note about Gender, Sexual Orientation, and Language

This book is written primarily for people at risk of unintended pregnancy and the people who care about them. The vast majority of those at-risk people are cisgender, female-identified, heterosexual girls and women. For this reason I use the words "girl" and "woman" throughout.

The terms "girl" and "woman" define *gender*, which is an inner sense of self that about 96 percent of people who menstruate have. I may use the terms "women" and "girls," but this book is for *anyone* who can benefit from it. Transgender and nonbinary people need health care information that is accessible to them, so I take an additive approach. Readers will find the gender-neutral words "person," "people," and "folks" in the book as well and, at times, "people with uteruses" or "people who menstruate."

This book has a large focus on pregnancy prevention, contraception, and unintended pregnancy. The sexual activity that results in unintended pregnancy is penis-in-vagina sex, so you will notice this book focuses largely on safety and health around that type of sex. People of any sexual orientation and gender can have penis-in-vagina sex, so the information is relevant to any-one with any sexual orientation who has a uterus or is in rela-tionship with someone with a uterus.

The chapters on the menstrual cycle; STIs; sexual pleasure; and agency, boundaries, and consent are relevant to all people regardless of sexual orientation or gender. There is a section on safe queer sex in the chapter on STIs.

1

Your Menstrual Cycle

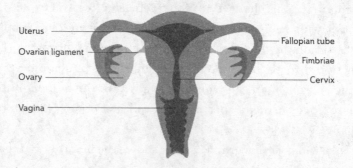

Uterus — Fallopian tube
Ovarian ligament — Fimbriae
Ovary — Cervix
Vagina

D id you know that from the time of your first period until you reach menopause in your late 40s or 50s, your body prepares for pregnancy every single month? The cycle of changes your body goes through lasts for the entire month. Your actual period is just the final phase of it. If you don't get pregnant during a month, the period is what cleans out everything so your body can do it all over again. If you did get pregnant, your period would not come, which is why missing a period is the first sign of a pregnancy.

To understand how birth control works, you first need to understand how your body works. That is why we start with an explanation of your menstrual cycle. This chapter will raise your awareness of how your body functions and give you an appreciation for just how remarkable a female body is. *Your body* is.

The monthly cycle can be broken down into four phases. Let's take a look at them.

Your Menstrual Month

The female "sex hormones" estrogen and progesterone are the main players in this monthlong cycle. They are responsible for many of the changes in your reproductive tract and also impact your energy, your moods, and your sexual moods. Follicle-stimulating hormone (FSH) and luteinizing hormone (LH) function directly on the ovaries, facilitating ovulation, which is the release of an egg from the ovary into the fallopian tube, where your partner's sperm can reach it and a pregnancy can be conceived.

Take a look at this graph, which shows the monthly swings of all four of these hormones.

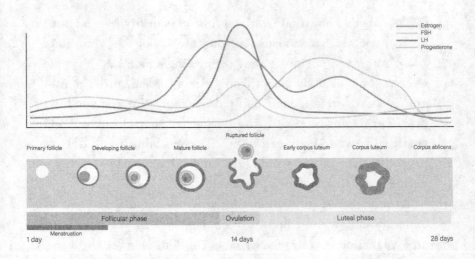

Now we will look at each of the four phases.

1. Follicular Phase (approximately days 7–12 of your cycle)

While medical professionals count the first day of your period as "day 1" of your cycle, the physiologic new cycle begins at the *end* of the period, around day 6 or 7. During the week after your period, your body begins its monthly preparation for conception. We call this week the follicular phase because FSH stimulates the ovaries to make them produce estrogen and progesterone. A fresh uterine lining begins thickening inside your uterus. Most women feel good during this week, as the symptoms of the period have ended and circulating sex hormones, estrogen and progesterone, increase as they get closer to ovulation. Energy for projects, exercise, and activities is bountiful. If each phase was compared to a season, this follicular phase is the *springtime* of your month.

2. Ovulatory Phase (days 13–19)

This phase begins one to two days before ovulation, the process in which your ovary releases a mature egg into the fallopian tube. This phase ends a few days after ovulation. This is your *fertile* week. (Fact: You are only fertile for one week of every month, but unless you are paying very close attention, it is hard to know exactly when that is.) If there is semen in your vagina and reproductive tract during this phase, you are likely to conceive a pregnancy. A spike in LH causes ovulation. Your estrogen and testosterone are at their monthly peak, which causes many women to feel sexy, in the mood, and easily turned on. It's a great time to go dancing, express yourself, be out and about. You can see it as your monthly *summer*, when you have extra radiance and energy. If you use a barrier method as your birth control, this is the week to be *extra* careful with it to avoid a pregnancy.

Cool Fact: During ovulation, your cervix produces a slippery mucus that resembles egg whites. This is your fertile mucus. You may notice it on your toilet paper when you wipe in the morning or just feel more wet than usual in your vagina. If you could look at it under a microscope, you would see that it contains sugar-coated ladders. Sperm use these ladders to climb through your cervix and get to the egg you just released, snacking on the sugar for energy along the way.

Rumor: I think something is wrong with me. I feel a pain on the side of my lower belly in the middle of my month, right between my periods. It doesn't last long, but I notice it almost every month.

Fact: Some women feel a sensation of pain when the egg is released during ovulation. The name for this is *mittelschmerz*, and it is normal.

3. Luteal Phase (days 20–28 or whenever your period starts)

This is the beginning of the cycle's end. If the egg your ovary released did not get fertilized, estrogen and progesterone levels begin a downward slide this week. This hormonal change causes your body to prepare to menstruate, to slough off the uterine lining not needed to support a pregnancy. As your sex hormone levels fall, you may experience the symptoms of premenstrual syndrome (PMS). This usually starts in the second half of this phase as you approach your menses. Symptoms may include headache, breast tenderness, bloating, sugar cravings, irritability, moodiness, and fatigue. Things that may help decrease these symptoms are exercise, time in nature, extra sleep and other forms of rest, vitamin E supplements, and essential fatty acids, including evening primrose oil or flaxseed oil. These supplements are particularly good for your reproductive tract. The luteal phase is the *autumn* of your month.

Cool Fact: Emotional honesty. During the week before your period, are you easily angered and irritated by certain people? Do you write it off as "just PMS"? Consider this: A wise friend once told me that during this week, a woman is more emotionally truthful and cannot pretend things are fine when they are not. During the week before your period, it's harder to tolerate things that don't feel right to you. Maybe it's worth examining your irritation and reflecting about whether you have been putting up with things you should not be.

Rumor: I just have to live with the depression I get the week before my period each month. I stay alone in my room, I hardly eat, and sometimes I feel so hopeless about everything that I have thoughts of self-harm. This is just PMS though, right? So there is nothing that can be done about it?

Fact: Some women experience mental health changes severe enough during the premenstrual week that they need treatment.

It is *not* normal to isolate, self-harm, or have thoughts of suicide as part of your monthly cycle. If this happens to you, you may have Premenstrual Dysphoric Disorder (PMDD), which can be treated by a psychologist or mental health professional. PMDD may be treated with counseling, hormonal birth control, an antidepressant, or a combination of these. It will not go away on its own and you deserve a life free of these difficulties, so go ahead and seek help. Please see the resources at the end of this chapter.

4. Menstrual Phase (days 1–6 of your period)

When your hormone levels fall to the lowest levels of your month, menstrual bleeding begins. These low hormone levels cause your uterus to shed its lining, which was made to hold and nourish a fertilized egg (the start of a pregnancy). Your cervix drops and opens a little bit to let the blood out, and this opening is accompanied by cramping for many women. Some women feel lower back pain and have either loose stools or constipation and other bodily symptoms, especially for the first couple of days of the menses, which are usually the heaviest. After the heavy bleeding days, you will lightly bleed or "spot" until the uterus is cleaned out. Then the whole cycle begins again, your hormone levels start rising, and the follicular phase of building a fresh lining and preparing to release an egg starts again.

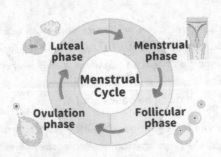

Coping with Your Period

Is your period an unwelcome, uncomfortable monthly hassle? If so, consider reframing it to look at it in a different way. What if you saw your menstrual days as your *inner winter*, a time to slow down the pace of your activities and prioritize rest and self-care? What if you used those days of heavy bleeding as a chance to relax, treat yourself, and recharge your batteries for the month ahead?

To soothe cramps and menstrual pain, eat warm foods, drink herbal tea with honey, use a heating pad, and take ibuprofen every four to six hours for cramps as needed. To practice self-care that honors your body during its menses, play relaxing spa music in your room, light a red candle, enjoy dark chocolate, take a break from social media, and read an inspiring book. If you watch shows, keep them funny or uplifting. Use your rest time to write letters or reach out to friends or relatives for a phone chat. Paint your nails or give yourself a home facial. Journal about intentions for the month ahead. Remember, resting during your menses is actually healthy for you.

In earlier times, many premodern cultures had special places, called menstrual huts or tents, for women to rest during their periods. This concept was popularized by a book called *The Red Tent*, a story about women in ancient Israel. The author theorized that menstrual huts or red tents were history's first version of a spa for women, where they could receive a massage, take a break from hard work, drink medicinal teas, and hang out with their friends while they were on their periods. In some circles, modern women are reclaiming this type of tradition, creating their own red tents with the idea of building rest, relaxation, and self-care into their monthly schedule.

Have you noticed that women living close to each other tend

to all get their periods at the same time? How cool would it be if they could all go hang out and rest at a spa together for those days? Some forward-thinking companies are even giving women paid days off for their menses. Life as a high school student does not easily lend itself to following this kind of routine, but can you think of ways to take care of your body during your period?

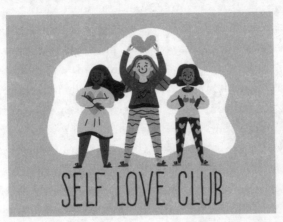

Should I get my period every 28 days?

Most women have a period that comes once a month, more or less. But there can be a lot of variation to cycle length, and these variations are all normal. Some people get a period every three weeks, or every four and a half or five weeks. Most women's cycles last between 26 and 31 days. That means, it is 26 to 31 days from the first day of your period to the first day of your next period. The period itself lasts, on average, from four to eight days. Less than a quarter of all women actually menstruate exactly every 28 days, so don't worry if your cycle is shorter or longer than that. And, if your period has always been irregular, then that is normal for you! Stress, excessive exercise, lifestyle changes, and travel can all impact the hormone levels of your body and change your period's schedule.

I am an athlete. Should I be doing my regular training during my period?

Everyone's body is different, and everyone's period is different. For some women, exercise eases the symptoms of cramping and bloating. It is fine to listen to your body and exercise if it feels right for you. The only real exception to this is doing inversions. According to the wisdom of traditional Ayurvedic and Chinese medicines, it is best not to be upside down while on your period. If you're a gymnast, dancer, cheerleader, or practice yoga, consider skipping inversions, positions in which your abdomen/pelvis is above your head, on the especially heavy days of your period. It makes sense to let gravity help the blood and tissue flow out of your body.

Teenagers often experience heavy periods and significant cramping during the first couple of years of menstruation. During this time of life, your body is working extra hard to figure out how to menstruate, and it can be intense. If your periods are hard to manage, I invite you to really consider taking those days of rest and be gentle with yourself. There will be plenty of time to be active during the rest of the month.

What about sex during my period?

Just like with exercise, some women feel fine about having sex during their period, and some prefer not to. Having sex during your period won't harm anything, but how you feel about it is really up to you.

We have just learned about how the hormones in your body do something different every single day of the month as your body prepares for ovulation, releases the egg, and, if not fertilized, prepares to and then sheds the uterine lining with a period. These constantly changing hormones do not just affect your uterus and ovaries—they influence other things too—your moods, energy levels, sex drive, appetites, and what you feel like focusing on.

One way to get more in tune with your body as it changes through the month is to observe and track these changes with a cycle-tracking app or menstrual awareness journal. When you track the shifts you notice, you can tailor your routines and activities to be in sync with your cycle. And you will be less likely to be caught unprepared for a period. Tracking your period can also alert you to a missed period so you can find out if you're pregnant right away. Some cycle-tracking apps are:

* For general use: Flo, a popular app with a simple user interface
* For gender-neutral tracking: Clue, a reliable, simple tracker
* Designed just for teen and tween girls: MagicGirl
* Recommended for folks with irregular periods: Life

Rumor: I don't get periods every month. My period is irregular, and I only get between three and five a year. My mother and her sister, my aunt, are the same way; it seems to run in our family. I don't need birth control because, with such irregular cycles, I don't think I can get pregnant.

Fact: Some women do not have monthly periods but have them irregularly and infrequently. If that is the case for you, then that is *normal* for you. There can be many underlying reasons why, such as genetic differences that run in your family. For example, some women have a hormonal profile with a variation in the balance of estrogen and testosterone. The medical community calls this hormonal variation polycystic ovarian syndrome (PCOS) because these hormonal differences also cause benign cysts on the ovaries that can be seen on ultrasound. It sounds a lot scarier than it is because, again, it's a variation that is normal for your body. If you are worried, you can be evaluated by a health care provider for your irregular periods. But don't be surprised if doctors cannot find the cause. In the meantime, you can get pregnant even if you have rare and irregular periods. I mean, you said that your mother has irregular periods too, and you got here somehow, didn't you?

Journal Prompts/Reflections

Journaling is a way to sort through and process new information or experiences. I am going to include journal prompts at the end of some chapters. If writing your thoughts down appeals to you, grab a notebook and a pen, and here you go:

* What is the story of your first period? Where were you, what happened, who helped you, what did you feel?
* Do you get PMS? What does that look like for you? Do you find yourself easily angered by anyone in particular during the week before your period? Reflect on issues that you are keeping inside to avoid problems or conflict with that person.
* What are some ways you could take extra-good care of yourself while on your period?

Further Resources

Premenstrual Dysphoric Disorder (PMDD)

International Association for Premenstrual Disorders (iapmd
.org/i-think-i-have-pmdd; iapmd.org/peer-support)

Me v PMDD symptom tracker app (mevpmdd.com)

Menstruation

Menstrupedia, an informative website with articles about
puberty, reproductive health, and menstruation, catered
specifically to teens and tweens (www.menstrupedia.com)

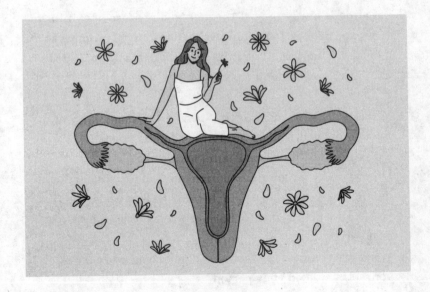

2

Birth Control Basics

*"We want far better reasons for having children than
not knowing how to prevent them."*
—*Dora Winifred Russell*

My town is a midsized college town well known for
beautiful rivers, hot summers, and a tradition of
large college parties. It sits in a valley three hours
north of San Francisco. If you head down a quiet side street
that runs beside a creek, park in the shady parking lot across
from the police station, and take the first flight of stairs, you
will arrive at a feminist health clinic that has provided free
and low-cost services to the community for over 45 years.
This clinic is where I have spent my days for the past six years.
The clinic has five exam rooms and a few alcoves where the
other clinicians and I sit and do our computer charting. My
alcove has a big window overlooking the street, so I can watch
the sky change throughout the day. The sky is usually bright
blue in sunny California, but I love to watch seasonal rain-
storms roll in and colorful winter sunsets. In the summer, I
sometimes watch wildfire smoke roll in and cover our skies.
Not my favorite.

I like to dress in bright colors when I come to work. I always wear big beaded earrings or a flashy necklace, something to add sparkle. I wear a white lab coat over my outfit anyway, which signifies my role as the care provider. I introduce myself to new patients as Dena and explain that I am a nurse-midwife. The vibe is casual, one person assisting another. Most of my visits here have to do with the things this book is about: birth control, problems with periods, STIs and other vaginal infections, the possibility of pregnancy. Often the purpose of the visit is something simple, like a refill of birth control. But once I am in the room with a person, I end up hearing about a lot of other things too. Because everything is interrelated with our bodies and our lives, isn't it? I have learned so much from all my clients over the years, and now I can share what I know with you.

Let's see who is on the family planning checkup schedule today. I have made up all the names and specific details of each person, but the medical facts are based on real-life situations.

Maisie is a high school junior who has a serious boyfriend. Her mother brought her into the clinic a year ago, concerned that she was at risk of getting pregnant. Maisie tried the Nuva-Ring and liked it. She appreciates the convenience of only having to remember once a month, and she likes the option of skipping periods, which she does for three out of every four months. Because her mother knows she is on it, she doesn't have to hide anything. She can store her rings safely in a brown bag in the family's refrigerator. It's no big deal.

Naomi is a teenager who started birth control pills a year ago to help with her painful periods. She set an alarm on her phone so she remembers to take it every day. Now she has a boyfriend and is thinking about becoming sexually active. She is glad she is already on the pill and protected. Naomi plans to stay on the pill for the next year and comes in today for her check-in and refill.

Jenna is a bisexual, polyamorous recent college graduate who uses condoms for their birth control. With their nonmonogamous lifestyle, they know they need the condoms for STI protection and feel if they are relying on them for birth control as well, they are certain to use them every time.

Kayla is a teen mother who had a baby 18 months ago. She works full time at an auto parts store after finishing high school through a continuation program. Kayla is on Depo-Provera. She comes in every three months for her shot. As a young working mother, she likes the convenience of not having to remember her birth control every day. She also is happy to skip having a period, which is a common side effect of Depo. Kayla feels that the shot makes it easy for her to stay on top of preventing another pregnancy.

Mieke is a varsity track athlete in her senior year of high school. She has track practice every day for several hours and, on top of that, is applying to colleges. She got a Paragard IUD because she wanted something that was very effective and easy to use. She loves that it is nonhormonal. Her periods have always been relatively easy, and she did not want to take hormones that would change them. Plus, this way, there is nothing that her parents can "find" and freak out about.

Candace is working her first job in marketing and got pregnant while on the pill. She forgot to bring them on vacation and missed several days of them. When she got home, she saw her boyfriend and had unprotected sex. She had ovulated during the days she missed her pills and got pregnant. Candace had an abortion a month ago and comes in today for her follow-up exam and an insertion of Nexplanon, a contraceptive implant that works for three years.

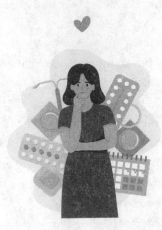

Condoms, ring, pill, shot, implant, IUD—there is quite a menu of birth control options these days. I am going to explain the available methods in the chapters ahead. And I am going to be realistic about what it is really like to use them, discussing both the *advantages* and *disadvantages* of each method. Because, let's face it, every single one has both.

There is no one perfect form of birth control that works 100 percent of the time for everyone with zero side effects. (Believe me, I wish there were.) The question is, which methods affect you in ways that are workable, which method is the best for *you*? Everyone's body is different, and everybody's needs are different. That's why it's good that there are choices here. It may take trying a few different methods before you find one that you like enough to stick with for a while.

When I start people on birth control at my clinic, I tell them to see it as the start of their birth control *journey*. I usually start someone with three months' worth of birth control and then have them come back and check in about how it's going. If it's going well, then they continue. If not, scrap that and on to the next one. But don't give up just because you tried one and didn't like it!

One of the defining differences between methods is that some are nonhormonal and some are hormonal. Nonhormonal means what it sounds like: They have no hormones in them, so your menstrual cycle, which we discussed in the previous chapter, does not change while you use the method. Nonhormonal methods include:

* Barrier methods, which are condoms, female/internal condoms, and diaphragms
* The Paragard, or copper, IUD

Hormonal methods work by altering your menstrual cycle so you don't ovulate and release an egg that can be fertilized. Within the category of hormonal methods, there are two subcategories. There are methods that combine estrogen and progestin (synthetic progesterone), which include:

* The birth control pill
* The patch
* The vaginal ring

There are also progestin-only methods:

* The Depo-Provera injection (the shot)
* The minipill
* The Nexplanon implant
* Several IUDs, including Mirena, Skyla, Liletta, and Kyleena

And then there are emergency contraceptive pills: Plan B, ella, Next Choice, etc.

Now let's look at a couple of common rumors about birth control and then the facts.

Rumor: I've already had sex a bunch of times without using anything. Don't you think it means I can't get pregnant?

Fact: Approximately 90 percent of young women (under 25) who are not using birth control will get pregnant within a year, according to research consolidated by the UCSF Bixby Center for Global Reproductive Health. Despite this fact, many women imagine that they might be infertile just because they have been lucky *so far*. But the deal is, if you have a uterus and you get periods, you should assume that you can get pregnant, and you very likely will if you are not on birth control.

Rumor: Birth control is bad for you because it has artificial hormones in it, so you shouldn't take it.

Fact: Birth control does have synthetic hormones in it, but that doesn't necessarily make it bad for you. And saying something like "it's bad for you" requires looking at what makes something *bad*. This brings us to the concepts of *risk* and *benefit*, which are how medical scientists and clinicians discern what is safe for you and what is not.

Anything you do has risks and benefits. Whenever you get in a car, there is a risk of being in a motor vehicle accident. You probably know someone who has. But the benefit of *getting where you need to go* outweighs the risk of an accident. Statistically, you are likely to get where you are going safely, although if you are in a car accident, it could be catastrophic. So you see, we are making risk/benefit decisions all the time. Every medication in existence, even Tylenol, has risks and possible side effects. The question is, do the benefits outweigh the risks? Birth control methods definitely have side effects and risks, which I will share with you in detail in the next chapters.

Before we do that, I want you to consider this: Any discussion of the risks of birth control needs to include the other side of the equation: the risk of being sexually active and not using birth control. Carrying a pregnancy to term and giving birth has significant risks to the pregnant/birthing person, a fact that is not talked about very often. Pregnancy and birth in the United States is significantly riskier for Black women and people of color. While you might know that common side effects of hormonal birth control can include nausea, breast tenderness, mood swings, and a changed period, did you also know that these are *all* normal symptoms of pregnancy? With birth control, stopping the method will reverse the side effects. With pregnancy, the only thing that will do that is terminating the pregnancy or giving birth.

Giving birth has risks and potential complications: protracted labor, bleeding and hemorrhage, vaginal tears, and even death. One out of five teen mothers in America will have a cesarean section delivery, which is major abdominal surgery and carries many risks. And of course, the life-changing task of parenting a child if you were not prepared or wanting to take on that responsibility.... I share this information not to scare you but to be realistic and to help you put things in *perspective*.

Things to consider when choosing a birth control method are your health, your lifestyle, and how frequently you have sex or will be having sex. Of course, the most important factor to consider is *how effective is it at preventing pregnancy*? This question is especially relevant for teens and young adults since youth is strongly associated with fertility.

Here is the thing about birth control: When methods are tested in clinical trials under medical supervision, they all are highly effective at preventing pregnancy. However, in real life with real people who are not enrolled in clinical trials, many of them are less effective than the research data suggests. We call this difference *perfect-use effectiveness* versus *typical-use effectiveness*. In other words, some birth control methods have more room for error than others, and this can significantly impact how well they work.

Below is a chart that shows which methods, in real-world, typical use, are pretty effective, really effective, and highly effective. Each of the next three chapters will discuss one row of the chart.

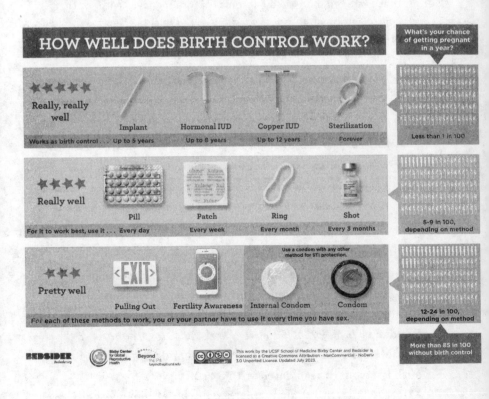

HOW WELL DOES BIRTH CONTROL WORK?

What's your chance of getting pregnant in a year?

★★★★ **Really, really well**

Implant — Up to 5 years
Hormonal IUD — Up to 8 years
Copper IUD — Up to 12 years
Sterilization — Forever

Works as birth control . . . Up to 5 years

Less than 1 in 100

★★★★ **Really well**

Pill — Every day
Patch — Every week
Ring — Every month
Shot — Every 3 months

For it to work best, use it . . . Every day

5-9 in 100, depending on method

★★★ **Pretty well**

Pulling Out
Fertility Awareness
Internal Condom
Condom — Use a condom with any other method for STI protection.

For each of these methods to work, you or your partner have to use it every time you have sex.

12-24 in 100, depending on method

More than 85 in 100 without birth control

Last Words: Definitions

Effectiveness: I am only going to discuss typical-use effectiveness, and I am going to call it real-life effectiveness since you, my reader, are a real person living a real life and not a part of a clinical trial in which medical personnel are making sure you use everything correctly every time you have sex.

Have Sex, Sexual Intercourse: I want to be really clear about what I am talking about when I say "have sex" or "sexual intercourse." There are many ways people can be physically intimate and sexual, but only one of those can cause a pregnancy. Oral sex, anal sex, making out, and hand jobs are examples of sex acts that will not result in a pregnancy. Only penetrative, penis-in-vagina sex can cause pregnancy. So in the following chapters on birth control, when I mention sex or sexual intercourse, I am referring to penis-in-vagina sex.

You: This information is for everybody with a body. However, when I say "you" in this book, I am referring to a person with a uterus.

Party-Ready: I am not condoning underage drinking or any recreational drug use in this book, but I am being realistic. Working with teens and young adults is my job, so I know that young people drink and use substances, and that when they do, it is not uncommon that they will also have sex. We all know that alcohol affects judgment, coordination, and capacity for clear thinking. So I will mention how well each form of birth control works if there has been drinking/substance use, and I will refer to this as its level of being **party-ready**.

Let's go.

Journal Prompts/Reflections

* Which birth control methods have you heard about that you think might be good ones to try?
* Which birth control methods have you heard about that sound scary or unappealing?
* If you have already used birth control, write about your experience with it.
* Do you worry about getting pregnant? If so, when do those worries come up? How much do they affect you? Any thoughts about what you would do if you got pregnant?

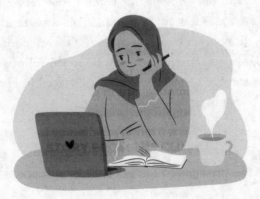

Further Resources

Bedsider (www.bedsider.org/birth-control): This site is great for side-by-side comparisons of all the methods.

Planned Parenthood (www.plannedparenthood.org/learn/birth-control): Planned Parenthood provides up-to-date and easy-to-understand information on all things contraception and reproductive health.

3

Methods That Work Pretty Well

Condoms, Barriers, Withdrawal, and Fertility Awareness

With the following methods, action needs to be taken to protect yourself every time you have sexual intercourse. Because there is a lot of room for forgetting and other errors, between 12 and 24 out of 100 healthy young women relying on these methods will get pregnant in a year. What follows is the information you need to use these methods correctly. With both motivation and consistency, these methods can be very effective, but that depends on *you*. On the plus side, they are nonhormonal and do nothing to and for your body except when you are actually having sex. Let's take a look at them.

The Condom

Condoms are a category of their own because they do double duty—they protect a person from pregnancy *and* STIs, and they are the *only* birth control method that does that. They literally make a barrier from infection between you and your partner (which will be further discussed in chapter 7, on STIs). As early as ancient Rome, condoms made of animal bladders were used for STI protection.

When used correctly, meaning used *every single time* you have sex (and remember, by this I mean penetrative penis-in-vagina sex), they are 98 percent effective at preventing pregnancy. Extremely effective! On top of that, there are no side effects or hormones, and you only need to use them while having sex versus taking a pill every day or having an IUD in place all the time. Plus they can even protect you from some sex-associated forms of vaginal infections, such as bacterial vaginosis (BV). One would think these contraception queens are a slam dunk birth control winner. Unfortunately, in real-world use, women often have a much different experience. Let's look at why that may be.

* Your partner must be as invested in protecting you from pregnancy as you are because their use lies mainly in his hands, so to speak.
* They need to be kept on hand and available.
* Because they are put on when sex takes place, brain changes from alcohol use and other recreational substances are obstacles to using them.
* They must be used every single time, even if you and your partner are long term and monogamous.

Effectiveness
In real-life use: 87 percent

Advantages
* Protect you from STIs
* Highly effective if used every time

* No hormonal side effects
* Only needed when actually having sex

Disadvantages

* Condoms place your body and safety in the hands of your partner.
* They must be thought about and available in the heat of the moment.
* *Condoms are not party-ready.* When there has been drinking or partying prior to sex, people are at risk of forgetting to use them.
* It is recommended that condoms are used *in addition* to another method of birth control. Then they are there as STI protection and an added layer of pregnancy prevention.
* If condoms are your preferred method of contraception, you should have an emergency contraception pill (ECP) available as a backup method. Take the ECP the next day if there is any doubt about whether condoms were correctly or completely used during sex. If you find yourself taking morning-after pills or ECPs more than once a month, you really need to consider adding another method of birth control, as ECPs should not be used more frequently than that.
* You are mostly likely to have success with condoms as your single birth control method if:
  * You have a committed partner who is actively involved in family-planning efforts. This would be a partner who comes with you to your clinic, purchases condoms, and shows genuine, ongoing interest in your health and pregnancy status.
  * You don't drink alcohol or use other substances prior to having sex.

- You don't have sex very often and tend to plan for it when you do.
- You *refuse* to have sex without a condom, *always* have condoms with you in your purse, handbag, or backpack, and you keep your eye on things to make sure your partners put them on and then keep them on.
- You keep emergency contraception on hand in case a condom breaks, slips off, or there is some other operator error.

HOW TO USE A CONDOM

1. Check that the condom hasn't expired—there will be an expiration date on the package.

2. Open the package carefully, without using teeth or scissors, and pull out the condom.

3. Make sure the condom is ready to roll on the right way: The rim should be on the outside so it looks like a little hat, and it will unroll easily. You can unroll it a little bit before putting it on to make sure it's right side out. If you accidentally put a condom on inside out, do NOT flip it around and reuse it—get a new one.

4. Pinching the tip, place the condom on the head of the penis. Leave a little bit of space at the top to collect semen. Unroll the condom down the shaft of the penis. I recommend adding more lubricant to the outside of the condom once it is on.

5. Have sex.

6. After ejaculation, your partner should hold on to the base of the condom and pull the penis out of the vagina before it gets soft, or the condom will slip off while still inside you.

7.   Throw away the condom in the trash; do not flush it. Have
     a supply on hand because a new one needs to be used
     each time.

Considerations

Some people have an allergy to latex, but fortunately there are
plenty of non-latex condoms on the market.

There are ribbed, colored, and flavored condoms to make life
more interesting. These are all safe to use.

Some guys will tell you they can't use condoms because their
penises are too big. That is untrue—they can buy extra-large
condoms at any drugstore, so don't fall for that story.

Condoms are best used with a water-based lubricant. Without it, the condoms can feel dry, and they can rub and irritate
vaginal tissues. Pre-lubricated condoms may not have enough,
so it is a good idea to buy a bottle of water-based lubricant, such
as K-Y or Astroglide, and squirt a generous amount of lubricant
on the condom (once it is already on the penis) prior to penetration. Never use petroleum-based lubes, such as Vaseline or min-
eral oil, as these break down the condom material.

Want to get more empowered about condom use so you can
help your partner put it on? Practice on a banana!

Many family-planning clinics offer free condoms or dispense
a couple dozen at a time if that is your chosen method.

Beware of Stealthing

A college freshman, let's call her Beatrice, was the first client
who told me about *stealthing*. Beatrice came to the clinic to get
a morning-after pill. When I walked into the exam room, I could

tell she was upset by the way she squirmed in her chair and didn't look straight at me. After I reviewed her medical history, I gave her a Plan B. She swallowed the pill and then told me about what happened the night before. Her new beau, whom she had been seeing for a few weeks and thought she liked, took off the condom in the middle of having sex—*without telling her*. "Yeah," she said. "He always says he doesn't like the way condoms feel." Now, she said, she is worried about STIs and even a pregnancy. She was furious about it and intended to break things off with him immediately.

Men have complained that they "don't like the way condoms feel" since those ancient Roman times. There is nothing new about that. Beatrice had every right to be mad—what this guy had done was nonconsensual and is a form of sexual assault in the eyes of the law. Within a few months of Beatrice's visit, more young women reported similar experiences, and I came to understand that stealthing, or removing the condom during sex without a partner's consent, is now a *thing*.

Beatrice took her emergency contraceptive pill, left urine for an STI screen, broke up with the guy, and carried on. A few weeks later another patient told me that she and her boyfriend had been using condoms as their birth control for three or four months. Then one night, he pressured her to have sex without one. He told her, "If you won't have sex without condoms, I'll just have to go on Tinder and find someone who will." She gave in and had sex with him without the condom, got pregnant, and then had an abortion.

Bottom line: Just because a guy desires you as a sex partner does not mean he will take care of you. *You* take care of yourself. If you are not in a committed relationship with someone who has earned your trust, it is wise to use condoms for STI protection, but have another form of birth control onboard to protect you from pregnancy. If condoms are your method of birth control, evaluate your partner's attitude about using them, and watch for cues that he may not be a reliable condom user. Those signs might be complaining about using them, not keeping condoms on hand, trying to persuade you not to use them, telling you things such as he has never gotten a girl pregnant, or purposefully getting you intoxicated before having sex.

The Internal or Female Condom

The internal condom was designed to give women more control because it goes inside the vagina instead of over the penis. This condom has an inner and outer ring. The inner ring is pushed inside against your cervix, and the outer ring hangs out of the vagina. While some people report reduced sensation with the internal condom, others say the outer ring stimulates the clitoris during sex and increases pleasure. These are available for free in many clinics and health departments, or they can be purchased online and in drugstores. They are worth exploring if you have an interest.

Effectiveness
In real-life use: 77 percent effective

Advantages
* Barrier method, so no hormones
* Can be put in up to two hours prior to sex, so more party-ready than male condoms
* Gives you more control—can't stealth this one
* Protects you from most STIs
* Non-latex so can be used with a latex allergy

Disadvantages

* May feel bulky and reduce female sensation
* May make squeaking sounds
* Needs to be used every time to be effective
* Takes practice to get comfortable with using it correctly

HOW TO USE A FEMALE CONDOM

There is already lubricant on the internal condom, but you can add more on the outside of the closed end.

1. Get yourself situated as if you're going to put in a tampon. You can be sitting on the toilet with your legs apart, standing with one leg up on the toilet seat or a chair, or lying on your back on the bed with legs open.

2. Put your finger inside the condom and insert it like a tampon.

3. Push the ring as far into your vagina as it'll go, all the way to your cervix. Your cervix feels like a nose way up in the back of your vagina.

4. Pull out your finger and let the outer ring hang outside your vagina. (Yes, it'll look a little funny, but on the plus side, the outer ring helps keep the condom in place and helps protect you from STIs that are transferred through skin-to-skin contact.)

5. Have sex.

6. After ejaculation, squeeze the outer ring and twist it closed like a baggie so semen doesn't spill out.

7. Pull out the condom gently.

8. Throw it away in a trash can. Don't flush it down the toilet because it's bad for your plumbing.

9.   Put in a new one each time you have sex.

One final thing: no double-bagging! You might think using male condoms along with an internal condom doubles your protection. Not true: It would just make both more likely to tear.

Diaphragm

The diaphragm is the other nonhormonal barrier method available. It is a silicone dome that is inserted in the vagina to cover the cervix and prevent sperm from getting through. It must be used with a spermicide gel, which is placed in the dome prior to insertion. While you do need a prescription for the gel, the diaphragm can be purchased online and you no longer need to be "fitted" at a clinic. The Caya diaphragm is now one-size-fits-most.

Effectiveness
In real-life use: 82 percent

Advantages
* A barrier method, so it is nonhormonal
* You have control over its use; can be party-ready because you can put it in several hours before having sex
* Non-latex
* Needs to stay in for at least six hours after sex, so you can just go to sleep and deal with removing it the following morning
* Can be used with multiple sex acts; you just add more spermicide each time

Disadvantages

* It takes practice to get used to it, and you need to be comfortable putting your fingers deep inside your vagina.
* It needs to be cared for and maintained: washed, dried, and stored, and examined for cracks or tears before each use.
* Because there is so much to using it correctly, it has a real-life effectiveness rate of 82 percent. That means 18 out of 100 women using it for a year will get pregnant. Studies show that how much the user wants to avoid a pregnancy determines how successfully she will use it.

HOW TO USE A DIAPHRAGM

1. Wash your hands well with soap and water.

2. Check your diaphragm for holes and weak spots by holding it up to the bathroom light. Filling it with water is also a good way to check—if it leaks, you've got a hole, which defeats the whole purpose.

3. Put a teaspoon of spermicide in the cup and spread some around the rim too.

4. Get situated like you're going to put in a tampon.

5. Separate your labia with one hand, and use the other hand to pinch the rim of the diaphragm and fold it in half.

6. Put your index finger in the middle of the fold to get a good, firm grip. (And yes, you'll be touching the spermicide.)

7. Push the diaphragm as far up and back into your vagina as you can. Use your finger to sweep to the back to make sure your cervix is covered. Your cervix feels like the tip of a nose,

and the whole cervix should be behind the dome of the diaphragm.

Leave the diaphragm in for six hours after sex. If you have sex a second time, insert more spermicide. (Ortho Gynol II comes with an applicator that measures how much you'll need and gets it where it needs to go.) Then the six-hour clock starts again, counting from the last time you have sex.

HOW TO REMOVE A DIAPHRAGM

1. Wash your hands.

2. Insert your index finger inside your vagina and hook it over the top of the rim of the diaphragm.

3. Pull the diaphragm down and out.

4. After you take it out, wash it with mild soap and warm water. Let it air dry.

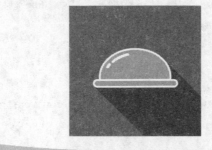

Withdrawal Method

Pulling out, or the pull-out method, is the oldest method known to humankind. This method is simple, nonhormonal, and cost-free, but its effectiveness lies *entirely* in the hands of your male partner. If he does it right, every time, it works well. But you

have no control at all, even though it is *you* who can get pregnant. Therefore, unless you would trust your partner with your
life or are open to getting pregnant, I do not recommend relying on the withdrawal method as your primary birth control. It
can be used in addition to another method to make a truly solid
contraception plan.

Effectiveness

In real-life use: 78 percent, which means about one in five
women using it will get pregnant in a year. Alcohol and recreational substance use plummet the chances that your guy will
pull out successfully, so it is not a method that is *party-ready*.

How to Do It

Your partner pulls his penis out of your vagina before he cums
and ejaculates on your belly, the bed, or anywhere away from
your vulva and vagina. That's it!

Considerations

It is better than nothing.

It has to be done correctly every time, so your partner cannot get lost in the moment, or have had drinks, or miscalculate,
or . . .

It is best to have an ECP on hand in case your partner doesn't
pull out in time.

There is also a small amount of semen present in precum,
so there is a slight risk of pregnancy even if he does pull out in
time.

Fertility Awareness

Fertility awareness, which is also called natural family planning, is the practice of tracking your body's daily changes in order to monitor for signs of impending ovulation, and then of ovulation itself. Practitioners of fertility awareness *abstain from sex* or use condoms during the fertile window around ovulation, from about two days before ovulation until five days after, so roughly seven days of every month. This method takes a commitment from both a woman and her partner, as well as a high level of organization and motivation to follow daily routines of monitoring and tracking symptoms. This is perfect for women in committed partnerships who enjoy observing and honoring their cycles and want to take that kind of observation to the next level. I have seen teens explore fertility awareness but not rely on it as their primary birth control. Someday, during a less transitional phase of life, these younger people may revisit it.

Effectiveness

In real-life use: Unclear. Various studies suggest it can be anywhere from 77 percent to 98 percent effective.

Advantages

* Nonhormonal
* No side effects
* Focuses on the subtle changes of a woman's body, which results in heightened body awareness and respect
* Can be used in reverse to help you when you do want to conceive a pregnancy

Disadvantages

* Requires *daily* tracking of symptoms and vaginal fluids over many months for a woman to develop the level of body knowledge she needs to do this correctly. Most women abstain from sex for about a week each month, and it's not your period week either.
* Many lifestyle factors, such as late nights, alcohol and drug use, irregular sleep schedules, working night shifts, and use of medications, can all impact your cycles and make accurate symptom tracking more challenging.

How to Do It

There are a number of ways to use fertility awareness, and the internet is full of books and classes to choose from. Most methods combine tracking your cycles, monitoring your daily cervical mucus (remember how I mentioned your slippery fertile mucus when you ovulate?), and measuring your basal body temperature, which is obtained with a specialized thermometer used the first thing in the morning to detect the tiny rise in body temperature that occurs right before ovulation.

For full instructions, it is best to get a book or workbook on the subject. One excellent choice is *Honoring Our Cycles: A Natural Family Planning Workbook* by Katie Singer.

Considerations

This method is best for someone who would be okay with a pregnancy if it happened. Some women use it to space out their children, tracking cycles between pregnancies. The symptoms are most reliable for people whose life routines, such as when they go to sleep and when they wake up, are consistent and don't change much from day to day.

Honorable Mentions

Spermicide

There are a number of spermicide products, including vaginal contraceptive films, spermicidal gels, a new gel called Phexxi that lowers the vaginal pH so sperm cannot thrive, and even a spermicide-filled foam sponge, currently off the market but possibly available again soon. All of them have a real-life effectiveness rate under 80 percent, which means more than 20 out of 100 women will get pregnant in a year when using spermicides as their birth control. This is just not effective enough to stand alone, but spermicides can be used *with* condoms for an effective, nonhormonal contraception plan.

Abstinence

The choice to *not* have penis-in-vagina sex is a 100 percent effective, nonhormonal, no-side-effect way to prevent pregnancy. However, it only works if you stick to it.

Advantages: No hormones, no side effects, no cost. Creates space for exploring the many other forms of sensual intimacy and pleasurable touch.

Disadvantages: Your partner(s) will need to be 100 percent on board with it and help you stick to it. This method is *not party-ready*, as drinking impairs your judgment and clarity. Abstinence and alcohol do not mix.

Stories from the Clinic

Melissa and her boyfriend, Jason, have been sexually active for about a year. They are each other's first sexual partners, and at first they used condoms every time. Lately, they use condoms sometimes and the withdrawal method sometimes. The inconsistency causes Melissa anxiety.

Melissa came to the clinic because she and Jason were tired of both the condoms and the worries. She wanted only nonhormonal options because she had been exploring fertility awareness and didn't want to change her cycles. She had pages of menstrual charts to show me, and she had been charting her cycles and cervical mucus for six months already.

I counseled her that fertility awareness is not as effective as other methods, so she should consider how she would feel about a pregnancy. She told me she did want to have a baby in a few years, but definitely not now. She decided to try a diaphragm, so I grabbed the sample diaphragm we keep sterile and ready at the clinic. I showed her how to use it and watched her put it in and take it out. She left with a prescription for Gynol II spermicide, available at any local pharmacy, and instructions on ordering the Caya diaphragm online. I also gave her a bag of condoms to use until her diaphragm came.

I had her come back in three months to see how it was going. When I saw her for the follow-up, she reported that she liked the diaphragm and that her boyfriend Jason helped her clean it and prepare it with the spermicide. She continued to track her cycles with the goal of eventually using the diaphragm only during her fertile window. But for now she was satisfied with her contraception plan.

Jade was a college freshman living away from home in a college dorm. Her lifestyle included nonmonogamous sex with both ongoing partners and occasional casual hookups. Jade used condoms for her birth control because they protected her from both STIs and pregnancy. Our clinic can dispense up to 36 free condoms and an emergency contraceptive pill once a month, and we saw her every month so she could get them.

"Women tell me that lately guys say they don't like condoms," I said to her one afternoon.

"Well, I had gonorrhea once a long time ago, and let me tell you, I never want another STI again," Jade said. "So if they try that on me, I just tell them to beat it."

Journal Prompts/Reflections

* Here is a situation: You are with a guy you really like, you are messing around, and things are getting hot and heavy. You are not on birth control and have used condoms with other partners in the past. You want to have sex with him, but now he says he doesn't want to use a condom because he doesn't like them. How would you insist that he wear a condom? Write down what you would say and read it aloud.

* Successful condom use requires preplanning. Where are some places you could keep condoms so they would be on hand if you needed them? Examples: bedside table, purse, backpack. (Okay, this was a trick question. Now put away the notebook and, if you have condoms already, put them in those places; if not, go buy some and do that.)

Further Resources

Caya diaphragm (for more information or to order online: www .caya.us.com)

4

Methods That Work Really Well—Part One

The Pill, the Patch, and the Ring

How does hormonal contraception prevent pregnancy?

Hormonal birth control works by stabilizing hormone levels in your body throughout your month, which pushes a *pause button* on your monthly ovulation cycle. Instead of the hormones rising and falling, everything stays on an even keel. You do not ovulate, and if you do not ovulate, then there is no egg available to be fertilized. Each method achieves this in a slightly different way, but the bottom line with all hormonal methods is that they give you a steady state of hormones instead of those spikes and dips we saw in the menstrual cycle chapter. Without those spikes and dips, you don't ovulate and your cervical mucus thickens so the sperm cannot get through. As soon as you stop taking them, it is like releasing the pause button—you ovulate and then have a period about two weeks later.

This means that when you go off birth control, you can get pregnant before you have a period, so be aware.

Hormonal birth control is very effective at preventing pregnancy but only if taken consistently. With perfect use, these methods are 99 percent effective at preventing pregnancy, but in real-life use they are all about 93 percent effective, which is still very effective. In this chapter, we will look at the three forms of birth control that contain a *combination* of estrogen and a progestin: the pill, patch, and ring.

But wait—taking hormones doesn't sound natural. Aren't these hormones bad for you?

There are only a few medical conditions, rare in young women and girls, that make the use of combination birth control risky. These include some forms of heart disease, high blood pressure, cancer, liver disease, a history of blood clots, or migraines with auras/vision changes. And if you are a smoker (meaning, you smoke at least half a pack of cigarettes per day), you should not use birth control with estrogen. Otherwise, birth control is safe for almost all women. And the progestin-only methods in the next chapter are safe to use, even for women who are smokers or have those above-mentioned medical conditions. Now, hormonal birth control *can* have side effects, and we will go over all those. Side effects are not usually dangerous, but they can be bothersome. Stopping use of the method resolves them.

When people talk about "natural," I like to consider what "natural" really means. So what *is* natural for women of reproductive age? Let's answer that question through an evolutionary biologist's lens. For all of human history, until between 50 and 80 years ago, most women were married off soon after puberty and had babies every couple of years from their teens into their 40s. It was *natural* and normal for women to have 8, 9, 11, heck, even 15 or more children! Ask your parents about their grandmothers—in your family, women may have had 10 or so babies only a couple of generations back. That, for most of human history, has been *natural*. Now, pregnancy and breastfeeding both push *pause buttons* on a person's monthly cycle (just like hormonal birth control does). So, if our great-grandmothers had 10 children, their cycles were paused for almost three years (nine months of pregnancy plus two years of breastfeeding) per baby. That means for 30 years of their 40 reproductive years they were *not* having periods. Bottom line: Most women throughout history did not have years and years of uninterrupted monthly periods.

Fast-forward to modern times, when young women go to school, have jobs, maybe plan for college and careers, and are less likely to get married while in their teens. Women nowadays have an average of two children, and it's not unusual to have only one or to be child-free by choice. Now, if these women never use hormonal birth control, they will have hundreds and hundreds of monthly menstrual cycles during their reproductive years, going through those changes every single month. Perhaps that is not truly *natural* either. Our lives have evolved faster than our biology has, and we really cannot say what is *natural* anymore. Better to consider what feels right *for you*.

Rumor: I heard that taking hormonal birth control can cause infertility or make it difficult to get pregnant when you want to.

Fact: Hormonal birth control has been around since 1960 and has been very well studied. There is *zero* association between using combination birth control and infertility or difficulties conceiving later. In fact many women conceive right away when they get off birth control, surprising themselves. When that pause button is released, as I mentioned above, the body jumps at the chance to ovulate.

The Pill, or Combination Oral Contraceptives

When people come to our clinic to get "birth control" for the first time, they often assume they will be getting birth control *pills*. Birth control pills, or oral contraceptives, were the first form of hormonal contraception available. They were approved for use in 1960, over 60 years ago! The other hormonal methods available today all came into use in the 1990s, early 2000s, and beyond. So the pill was truly the leader of the pack, and its use in the 1960s was heralded as a tool of women's sexual liberation, significantly untethering sex from pregnancy for the first time in human history.

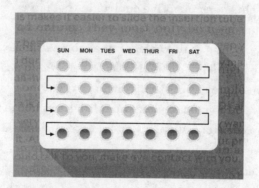

The pill is a tiny tablet that you take every day at the same time. In traditional pill packs, there are three weeks of hormone pills, a combination of estrogen and a progestin, that keep your hormone levels at a steady state, preventing ovulation and thickening cervical mucus. The last week of the pill pack consists of placebo pills, which you take anyway to keep the routine, and after a couple of days into the placebo pills, you get a period. When you finish your last pill of the pack, you start a new pack the very next day.

Nowadays, some pills are designed without that monthly placebo week, so women can skip their periods altogether or instead opt to have a period once every three months, which is four times a year.

Effectiveness
In real-life use: 93 percent

Advantages
* The pill is very effective if taken correctly.
* It can clear up acne for some women.
* The new low-dose formulations are well tolerated with few side effects.
* The pill puts contraceptive control in the hands of the woman taking them.
* There is nothing to do or see in the moment of sex—the medicine is already on board. Definitely *party-ready*.
* If you have side effects that you do not like, there is nothing to remove and you can just stop taking them. The hormones are completely out of your system within a couple of days of not taking them.
* Most women's periods get lighter, easier, and more regular while on birth control pills. That is one of their known side effects! In fact, the birth control pill is a common treatment for heavy, painful, or irregular periods. You can also choose to skip your period while on the pill by staying on the hormone pills continuously or for three months at a time, in which case you only have a period four times a year.
* They can be ordered through online telemedicine sites such as Nurx.com and can be stored at room temperature.

Disadvantages

* Taking a pill every day at the same time can be challenging.
* Some women have unpleasant side effects, which can include headaches, breast tenderness, dizziness, nausea, mood changes, and decreased sex drive.
* There can be rare complications of blood clots. Smoking and being over 35 both increase the risk of this. That is why this is not a good choice for smokers.
* The risks of vaping nicotine while using the pill has not been determined yet.
* They can cause irregular bleeding, especially if you are skipping periods on them.

How to Do It

The reason that pills work *pretty* well, instead of *very* well, is that you have to take them every single day at around the same time. To up your chances of success, consider what time of day would work best for you. Mornings, before school or work, work well for some people. But if you sleep in on weekends, you are going to be late taking your pill, and that would make them less effective. So the time of day needs to be the same no matter what—weekday, weekend, at work, school, or home. Some people take their pills at night when they brush their teeth. But again, if on the weekends those people stay out late or sleep over with friends, they might miss their pill. You see, it can be tricky to find the right time. Some girls take it at lunchtime, others take it at 5 PM, and for this schedule they carry their pills with them in their bag or purse at all times.

Set an alarm on your phone to remind you. (Set a couple, 20 minutes apart!) If you already take a daily medication, you will probably do just fine taking this one—and it can be taken with other medications. "On time," by the way, means within an hour of the scheduled time, so it can be an hour earlier or later and still be "on time."

How to Start Them

You can Sunday Start, which means you start your pills on the first Sunday after your next period begins. This syncs up your pill with your body's cycle and means you will never have your period on the weekend. Also, if you have been having unprotected sex, waiting until you have started your period ensures you are not already pregnant.

Or you can Quick Start—put the stickers that come with the pack across the top of your pills to match the day you are starting, and start today if you prefer. If you have already been having unprotected sex, take an at-home pregnancy test if you don't get a period during the placebo week.

HOW TO USE THEM

1. Take your pill every day at the time you have selected. Take them across from left to right, starting with the top row. Never take the pills out of order!

2. Use condoms for the first seven days of the first pack, as you are not yet protected until you have taken it for a week.

3. If you get nauseous, take it with food or right before bed.

4. If you miss a pill, take it as soon as you remember it, and then keep going at the regular time.

5. If you miss it altogether, double up the next day and use condoms if you have sex in the following seven days.

6. If you miss two pills, take two one day and two the next, and use condoms for the whole rest of the pack.

7. If you miss more than two pills, throw the pack away, use condoms, wait until you have a period, and then start all over again. If this happens again, you should probably try a different method, such as the patch or ring, which contain the same hormones but are an easier delivery system to use.

Considerations

You will need to store your pills somewhere, so they are hard to hide.

If you have never taken daily pills before, give yourself a three-month trial and see if you can get the hang of it. The first month will be the hardest. Use condoms for the following week any time you are not sure if you have taken your pills correctly. Make sure the days on the pill pack match the actual days of the week to prevent you from getting confused. It's wise to keep an emergency contraceptive pill on hand for backup too.

If you smoke half a pack of cigarettes or more a day, there are increased health risks with birth control pills.

If you notice major negative mood changes or you feel "crazy" on the pill, stop taking it and go see a health care provider. Some people experience significant mental health changes when they try the pill. It is unusual but serious.

Hormonal birth control works best when you stay on it consistently over time, so get your refills of pill packs before you run out. If you start and stop and restart pills, you can get spotting, irregular bleeding, and other problems. Taking pills inconsistently also makes an accidental pregnancy likely. *The most important pill to take on time is the first pill of a new pack, after the week of placebo pills.*

Estrogen in birth control can increase the risk of a blood clot, an extremely rare but dangerous condition. If you develop a red, tender, swollen lump in the calf, or experience chest pain, left shoulder numbness, or difficulty breathing, go to an ER immediately for evaluation. In a healthy young woman, blood clots are very rare, but you should still know the signs.

The Patch

The patch contains similar hormones to the pill but in a delivery system you only have to think about once a week. The patch is a very sticky adhesive patch that can be worn in four places: the outside of your upper arm, the back of your shoulder, your lower abdomen, or your buttock. You put a patch on once a week for three weeks, then have a patch-free week, which is like the placebo week on the pill, when you will have your period.

Cool Fact: Skin absorbs hormones very well. The hormone in the patch goes directly into your system via the skin instead of having to pass through your digestive system and liver first, like the pill. This may make it easier on your body over long-term use.

Effectiveness
In real-life use: 93 percent

Advantages
* You only have to remember once a week.
* Periods are very regular on the patch.

* You can choose to skip periods.
* It is woman-controlled and *party-ready*.
* It doesn't matter what time of day you change it as long as it's the patch change day.
* If you don't like it or have bad side effects, it is easy to just remove it; the hormones drop within a day.

Disadvantages

* It can be visible, especially if worn on the arm or shoulder, so you cannot easily hide this method.
* If you weigh more than 198 pounds or have a BMI over 30, it may not be as effective.
* It may cause estrogen-related side effects, such as nausea, bloating, tender breasts, or dizziness.
* It leaves a fuzzy outline on your skin that lasts a couple of days when you take it off.
* If you put it in the wrong place, it might not work.

HOW TO USE

There are four places the patch can be placed: the upper arm, the back of the shoulder, the abdomen below the belly button, and the butt cheek.

If you wait until your next period is over to start it, the patch will be synced up nicely with your own cycle and you will know you are not already pregnant. Or you can Quick Start it any day, then take a pregnancy test after two to three weeks to be sure you were not already pregnant when you started. Always use condoms for the first seven days of any hormonal method.

1. Your skin needs to be clean and dry, with no lotions, oils, perfumes, or products that would get in the way of it working.

2. Apply the patch as smoothly as possible, making sure the edges are firm against the skin. Press down for 10 seconds to make sure it sticks.

3. Change once a week on your patch change day—set an alarm to help you remember.

4. After three weeks, take one patch-free week. Your period will start on the second or third patch-free day.

5. Even if you are still bleeding, put on your new patch on the next patch change day.

6. You can skip the patch-free week and use the hormone continuously for three months before taking a patch-free week. However, if you do give yourself a monthly period, it will likely get lighter and easier over time. If you only have a period every three months, it may be a doozie.

7. Check your patch daily, especially after swimming or sports. If it comes off and it has been off less than 24 hours, put a new one on and keep going with your regular patch change day after that.

8. If it comes off and you don't know how long it has been off, use condoms with sex, wait until you have a period, and start a new four-week cycle toward the end of the period. Use condoms for the first patch week.

9. Fold the patch in half before you throw it away to keep the hormones contained.

10. Always use condoms for the first seven days when starting on the method.

11. Each week, put the new patch on a different spot of skin—some people go from butt cheek to butt cheek or side to side on the lower abdomen. The skin covered by the patch needs to breathe and recover!

Considerations

The patch is not safe to use if you smoke half a pack of cigarettes or more each day.

We don't know the risks associated with vaping and patch use.

Never put it on your breast!

Estrogen in birth control can increase the risk of a blood clot, an extremely rare but dangerous condition. Women over 35 or who are smokers are at increased risk. If you develop a red, tender, swollen lump in your calf; chest pain; left shoulder numbness; or difficulty breathing, go to an ER for evaluation. In a young, nonsmoking woman, blood clots are very rare, but you should still know the signs.

Vaginal Ring

The vaginal ring is a bendable, slim silicone ring that contains a combination of estrogen and a progestin, similar to the pill and the patch. Like the patch, the hormones are absorbed through the skin, but the ring is placed in the vagina, so the hormones go right where they need to be and no one can see it. To put it in, you squish the ring between your fingers and slide it into your vagina like a tampon. It stays in for three weeks if you want a period week, or four weeks if you prefer to skip your period. It is easy to use because you only need to think about it once or twice a month.

Effectiveness

In real-life use: 93 percent

Advantages

* The vaginal ring is easier to use than the pill or patch.
* It has a low rate of side effects. The vagina actually absorbs hormones so well that only a very small amount of hormone is used. Even if you experienced unpleasant side effects (e.g., nausea, headaches, breast tenderness, or moodiness) on the patch or pill, you may not have them with the vaginal ring.
* Some sex partners find that the soft ring is like ribbing for extra pleasure.
* It may clear up acne.
* Your period will likely get lighter and shorter over time. It is in and *party-ready*.

Disadvantages

* The rings should be stored in the refrigerator after four months, so it is harder to hide a stock of them at home. If you are on the move and don't have a fridge to keep them in, you can only keep a four-month supply at a time.
* Some sex partners may say they prefer that you take it out during sex. It can be out for an hour or two, and then you can rinse it in lukewarm water and reinsert it. But if you fall asleep and forget to put it back in afterward, you lose your protection from pregnancy. It is a better policy to keep it in at all times and tell partners they will learn to like it, as it is extra ribbing for their pleasure.
* The ring can have side effects: nausea, irregular bleeding, mood changes, etc.

HOW TO USE

If you wait until your next period is over to start it, the ring will sync with your own cycle and you will know you are not already pregnant. Or you can Quick Start it any day, then take a pregnancy test after two to three weeks to be sure you were not already pregnant when you started. Always use condoms for the first seven days of any hormonal method.

1. Squish the ring between your fingers and slide it into your vagina like a tampon. This is best accomplished sitting on the edge of the toilet with your legs open, standing up with one foot up on the toilet or a chair, or lying on the bed with knees bent and legs apart.

2. After it is as far back as it comfortably goes, slide your fingers out and the ring will open. If you can feel the rim at your vaginal opening, insert your finger and push that part of the ring up so it's tucked behind the pubic bone on the top of your vagina, just inside the opening. When it is in correctly, you will not feel it at all.

3. Leave in for three or four weeks.

4. After three weeks, remove it for exactly seven days, have a period, and then put in a new one even if you are still bleeding. To skip the period, remove and replace all at once in four weeks.

5. To remove: Insert a clean finger into your vagina just far enough to reach the closest rim, hook your finger on it, and gently pull it out. Throw it away in a trash can.

6. If it comes out or you take it out for some reason, rinse in lukewarm water and reinsert.

Considerations

Because it contains estrogen, it is not the best choice for smokers.

There is a 12-month ring called Annovera that was FDA approved in 2018 and may be available in some places. With that one, you can either leave it in for the full year or take it out for a week and then reinsert it each month to have a period.

Estrogen in birth control can increase the risk of a blood clot, an extremely rare but dangerous condition. If you develop a red, tender, swollen lump in your calf; chest pain; left shoulder numbness; or difficulty breathing, go to an ER for evaluation. In a young, healthy woman, blood clots are very rare, but you should still know the signs.

The vaginal ring cannot get lost—your vagina is closed at the back!

STORY FROM THE CLINIC

Kelsey was in high school and had been trying birth control pills on and off for almost a year. She forgot to take them a few times every month and then would have long bouts of heavy, irregular bleeding that always started after she missed pills. She was feeling drained and discouraged.

"Maybe hormones don't agree with me," she told me during her visit.

"Well," I said, "missing several pills each month certainly doesn't agree with you. That doesn't agree with anyone."

Kelsey had already had a couple of boyfriends, and even though she wasn't seeing anyone at the moment, she wanted to be prepared. I talked to her about her other options, and when I got to the vaginal ring, she made a face and said, "I don't want to put something in my vagina!"

We went over other options, such as the shot and implant, but she preferred to stick to the same hormones (combination estrogen and progestin) that were in pills. After I showed her the slim, flexible sample vaginal ring we keep in the room, she decided to go ahead and try the NuvaRing.

Kelsey's irregular bleeding stopped within two days of putting it in. She didn't feel it inside her, either, and at her three-month follow-up visit decided to continue on it. Fast-forward two years, and Kelsey went off to college with a year's supply of NuvaRing to tuck into her dorm room mini-fridge.

Journal Prompts/Reflections

* Write down your thoughts about taking hormonal birth control. What concerns do you have about it?
* If you have been on hormonal birth control in the past, or are using it now, describe how your body feels while using it.
* Of the methods described in this book so far, which ones might you consider? Why?

Further References

To order pills online, visit Nurx (nurx.com)

5

Methods That Work Really Well—Part Two

The Shot, the Minipill, and ECPs

The following options are progestin only. They do not contain estrogen and therefore have no increased risk of blood clots. Progestin-only birth control is safe for women with medical conditions that make taking estrogen risky. It is also safe for people who smoke and women over 35. The progestin in them suppresses ovulation and thickens the cervical mucus. Most of the progestin-only methods change your periods, which may become very light, sporadic, or disappear altogether while using them. This is because while on progestin-only birth control, your body does not make a thick uterine lining every month. If that lining isn't made, then there is nothing to shed with a period. Your normal period returns when you discontinue use.

The Shot

Also known as Depo-Provera, or "Depo," the shot is an injectable contraception that works for three months at a time. It is given rapidly into the gluteus maximus (butt muscle) or the deltoid muscle of the upper arm, and the injection is often almost painless. The shot is very easy to use and hide—the only thing you need to "keep" are your appointments four times a year. There is nothing to see, ask about, or take in or out. If you get your shots on time, the method is extremely effective at preventing pregnancy. Because it is progestin only, most people on it do not get regular periods or any period at all. The shot also has some notable side effects, which some people experience and some do not. Because of this, I have seen that people in my clinic either love it or dislike it.

Effectiveness
In real-life use: 96 percent

Advantages
* Easy to use—just come get a quick injection four times a year.
* Easy to hide—nothing to see, nothing to store, nothing to do. No "thing" is in you, like an IUD or implant. It is good for people who don't want anyone to know they are on birth control.
* *Party-ready*—nothing to do in the heat of the moment.
* After six months or so of using this method, 60 percent of users stop having periods. *Please understand: You will not have regular periods while using Depo.* Some women see this as an advantage and some do not.
* It is safe for almost all women, including smokers, women over 35, and women with heart conditions and other chronic diseases.

Disadvantages
* Needles—some people *hate* needles.
* It is common to have irregular spotting for the first few

months when starting Depo, and then, if you stick with it, the periods usually stop altogether. But those first three to six months can be annoying, with spotting and bleeding coming with no warning. Not everyone has this, but you won't know until you try it.

* You can't take it out once it is in, so it is a commitment to a three-month experience.

* Some women notice increased appetite, and there is an average five-pound weight gain in the first year of use. Not everyone gets this weight gain, but you won't know until you try.

* Other side effects can include moodiness, lower sex drive, acne, and bloating.

* This is the only method that is known to delay a return to ovulation after stopping use. It is not common, but in some people it can take up to nine months after discontinuing Depo to get regular cycles back. So if you think you might want to have a baby in the next year or so, this might not be the best option for you.

HOW TO USE

1. If you can, come for your first appointment when you are near or at the end of your period. This ensures you are not already pregnant and might decrease irregular spotting in the first couple of months.

2. Avoid unprotected sex (sex without a condom) for two weeks before the appointment. You will be given a pregnancy test (which is done by a urine sample, so you will be asked to pee in a cup) before you get your shot, but it takes two weeks between conception and a positive test. If you were pregnant

and you got the shot, it wouldn't harm the pregnancy, but it could mask the symptoms of the pregnancy, so you may not realize you are pregnant until you come in for your next shot.

3. A nurse or provider will give you the injection, either in your buttock (your biggest muscle) or the upper arm muscle (deltoid). It takes a couple of seconds.

4. That's it! Make sure you leave with an appointment card telling you when to come back in three months for your next one.

5. Use condoms for the first seven days of your first injection as backup. After that, your protection is continuous as long as you come back on time for subsequent shots.

Considerations

There is a concern that long-term Depo-Provera use may be associated with bone density loss during use. Because of this, Depo-Provera was given a black box warning in 2004, recommending that women use it for two years at a time and then take a break. In the 20 years since that warning was placed, there have not been any significant findings of disease related to this issue. The World Health Organization disagrees with the warning, and it eventually may be taken off the label, but in the United States, the warning still stands. At our clinic, we recommend that long-term Depo users take a calcium/magnesium supplement and try to get weight-bearing exercise to support bone health. We have not seen any specific medical issues with people's bones.

Rumor: Depo-Provera makes you gain weight. I know someone who gained 50 pounds on it!

Fact: Many medical studies have examined the association between weight gain and Depo-Provera use. And the verdict from data on thousands and thousands of Depo users is this: Women who gain weight with Depo use gain an average of five pounds in the first year of use. And after that first year, they don't really gain any more. For some people, gaining a few pounds can be healthy, helping them feel stronger and healthier. Other people may not want to gain weight. There is a big difference between five pounds and 50 pounds, so if someone has gained 50 pounds, it is certain that something is going on with them other than getting the shot.

The Minipill

The minipill, or progestin-only pill (POP), looks just like the regular birth control pill, except every single day is the same color. There is no placebo week. The minipill is "mini" because it is progestin only and does not contain estrogen, so there is a "mini" amount of hormone in it. Because of that, they are not as forgiving if you take them late or miss pills, which is the downside. But the upside is that it is a great option for women who cannot take estrogen (e.g., people who smoke or people with high blood pressure and other medical conditions). I have seen many women, including young ones, use it successfully when other methods did not work out. The minipill does not always make "the list" of birth control options, but that is about to change. In July 2023, the FDA approved it for OTC use—that is how safe it is! By summer of 2024 you should be able to buy it at your pharmacy *without a prescription!*

Effectiveness
In real-life use: 91 percent

Advantages
* Because it is a pill, it is not as big a commitment as the other progestin-only options, which include the shot, implant, and IUD. You can stop taking it at any time, and the hormones are gone from your system within a day or two.
* The minipill does not cause estrogen-related side effects, such as headaches, nausea, breast tenderness, or moodiness. It is safe for smokers and carries no increased risk of blood clots.
* Your period may get very light or disappear altogether while on this pill.
* You can use it if you want to *try* a progesterone-only method before moving to a long-acting one.
* It has a smaller amount of hormone than the shot does, so it is less likely to have side effects than Depo-Provera.
* It's good for people used to taking daily medications on a schedule.
* As long as you have been taking it at the same time every day, you are *party-ready*.
* The FDA has approved it for over-the-counter use, and it is the *first birth control pill* in the United States to have that status.

Disadvantages
* This pill is less forgiving if you are late taking it or miss a pill. If you take your pill three or more hours after the scheduled time, there is a possibility you will ovulate and

can get pregnant. It is advised to use condoms for a week after taking a minipill more than three hours late.

* It may cause irregular bleeding, especially if you are late taking it.

HOW TO USE

1. You can either start your pills on the first Sunday after your period begins to sync your pills to your body's cycles right away, or start them any day as long as you place the stickers across the top of your pills to make them match the day.

2. Take your pill every day at the time you have picked. Take them across from left to right, starting with the top row. Never take the pills out of order!

3. Use condoms for the first seven days of the first pack, as you are not yet protected until you have taken the pills for a week.

4. If you miss a pill, take it as soon as you remember, then keep going at the regular time. If you are more than three hours late taking it, use condoms for a week.

5. If you miss it altogether, double up the next day and use condoms as backup for a week.

6. If you miss two pills, take two one day and two the next, and use condoms for the whole rest of the pack.

7. If you miss more than two pills, throw the pack away, use condoms for birth control, wait until you have a period, and then start all over again. If this happens again, you should probably try a different method, such as the patch or ring, which have the same hormones but an easier delivery system.

Considerations

Hopefully I have made it clear that if there is any question about your missing pills or taking them late, use backup.

This is also known as the "breastfeeding pill" because it is safe for breastfeeding mothers. Progestin-only methods do not decrease a mother's milk supply, which estrogen might. It may actually increase milk supply.

Emergency Contraception Pills, or Morning-After Pills

ECPs are not considered stand-alone birth control but can be used after-the-act in case *something happens*. That *something* can be anything that resulted in possibly unprotected sex: You forgot to start your new pill pack, the vaginal ring slipped out, he took off the condom, you were drinking and forgot to use a condom. It is important to take one if you experienced nonconsensual sex or are the victim of sexual assault. (For more about sexual assault, see chapter 10.)

You can take a Plan B, Next Choice, My Way, or any other progestin ECP up to 72 hours (three days!) after unprotected sex, but it works best if you take it ASAP. This is why it got the nickname "the morning-after pill." Ella is a different form of ECP. Instead of containing a progestin, it has a medication that affects how progesterone is used in your body and can be taken up to *five days* after unprotected sex. *IUDs are also emergency contraception if placed within five days of unprotected sex*. More about that in the next chapter.

Using an ECP after unprotected sex decreases the chance of a pregnancy by 85 percent. ECPs work by stopping or delaying ovulation. They do *not* cause an abortion; they keep a pregnancy from happening in the first place. At our clinic we offer condoms and an ECP to anyone who comes through our door for anything because it is a good idea to have them handy for those just-in-case scenarios.

Advantages

* ECPs decrease the chance of a pregnancy by 85 percent after unprotected sex.
* Plan B and other levonorgestrel pills are available for purchase over the counter at pharmacies, drugstores, and some grocery stores.

Disadvantages

* ECPs are likely to cause irregular bleeding and may delay your period for up to a week.
* The progestin pills may not work as well for women weighing over 154 pounds. The Ella pill may be less effective for women over 198 pounds.

HOW TO USE

Take one pill as soon as possible after unprotected sex, up to 72 hours after with progestin pills (most of the brands are this kind) and up to five days after if the pill is an Ella. That is it!

Don't be alarmed if your period is late, but feel free to take a home pregnancy test two weeks after you take the ECP if you are worried.

Considerations

ECPs are for backup in case of an occasional *whoops*. They can be taken once a month, but they should not be used on the reg. If you find yourself taking an ECP once a month for three months in a row, I recommend that you evaluate your lifestyle and consider a different contraception plan.

Special Considerations: IUDs are also emergency contraception (see the following chapter for deets).

STORIES FROM THE CLINIC

Dierdre was a young client at our clinic who was living with many medical conditions. She had had heart disease since childhood and had already had two heart surgeries. She was an insulin-dependent diabetic, and she had severe asthma managed by several medications and frequent hospitalizations. She had a boyfriend and was sexually active. Because of her medical conditions, a pregnancy would be very risky for her. Dierdre used Depo-Provera because it was safe to use even with her health issues and because it was such effective and easy birth control.

Carrie tried several combination birth control pills and the NuvaRing, but she suffered from mood swings and nausea on all of them. Then she tried the progestin-only minipill and was thrilled to find that she experienced no side effects at all. She set an alarm on her phone and woke up early even on weekends to make sure she took it on time.

6

Methods That Work Really, Really Well

The Implant and IUDs

The methods in this chapter work really, really well because once they are in you don't need to do anything else, and you are protected from pregnancy for several years. The implant is 99.9 percent effective at preventing pregnancy, and the IUDs are all 99.2 percent effective at preventing pregnancy. That is as close to 100 percent as you can get without practicing sexual abstinence (not having penis-in-vagina sex). The methods in this chapter work for at least three years, and one IUD, the Paragard, provides protection for up to *twelve years*. And they are all reversible—you can have them removed at any time, with swift, complete return to your fertility. The upshot: If you want to be sexually active but do not want to get pregnant for the next few years, it is worth learning about these options.

The Nexplanon Implant

The Nexplanon is a small, bendable rod that is about the size of a match. It is inserted just under the skin along the inside of your upper arm, where it is almost invisible. It contains a slow-releasing progestin, which prevents ovulation and thickens cervical mucus while providing up to three years of contraception.

Putting it in is not a huge deal. It takes only a few minutes, and there is no pelvic exam required (unlike the IUD). It is a five-minute office procedure in which only your arm is touched. A numbing agent called lidocaine makes the insertion painless. These factors make it a good choice for people who are sexually inexperienced, modest, have a history of sexual trauma, or for whatever reason don't want their genitals touched by health care providers but still want highly effective contraception that will last a few years.

Effectiveness
In real-life use: 99.9 percent effective. That is highly effective!

Advantages
* The implant is private—it cannot be seen unless someone intentionally pokes on your arm to seek it out.
* Once it is in, there is nothing else to do. You are *party-ready* for three years.
* Many women stop having periods or have irregular, light periods on this method.
* If you like the method, you can remove and replace the implant in three years.
* The FDA may soon change the approval for use to up to four years instead of three.
* The method is safe for almost everybody and does not increase the risk of blood clots.
* There is a quick return to fertility after it is removed.

Disadvantages
* Because the implant is progestin only, it will change your period for the duration of its use. Most women have episodes of irregular bleeding or spotting for the first three to six months, then stop having periods altogether for a couple of

years. I list this as both an advantage and a disadvantage because some people love that side effect and some people do not.

* A few women experience irregular bleeding that does not stop after a couple of months. If this happens, you should return to the clinic where you got the implant for help. Your provider might give you a couple of packs of birth control pills to take. This usually stops the irregular bleeding and is safe. Consider trying that before giving up and removing the implant.

* Other side effects some women report are moodiness, depression, acne, a change in sex drive, and bloating.

* Your arm will be sore and may be mildly bruised for a couple of days after the insertion.

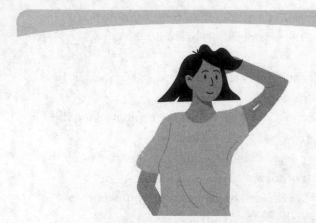

HOW THE IMPLANT IS INSERTED

1. For the two weeks before your insertion appointment, make sure to use condoms or another method so you are not already pregnant when you start.

2. When you come into the office, you will leave a urine sample in a cup for a pregnancy test.

3. You will be asked if you have an allergy to lidocaine, which will be used to numb your arm. If you have ever been numbed for a dental filling without complications, then you are likely not allergic to lidocaine.

4. You will lie on an exam table with your arm bent and resting by your head. The nurse or provider will use a tiny needle to inject a small amount of numbing medicine under the skin of your inner upper arm in the spot the implant will go in. This will cause a stinging sensation for about 30 seconds. Then the nurse will probably chat with you about this or that for a couple of minutes while the numbing takes effect.

5. The implant is so small it fits inside a needle. The nurse will slide this needle under the skin of your arm, which you won't feel because you will be numb there. Then she will push a button on the inserter that retracts the needle but leaves the implant in place. That whole process takes a few seconds.

6. It's in and you are done! The place where the implant went in is covered with tape and a gauze square, and a stretchy bandage is wrapped around your arm, with instructions to keep the bandage on for 24 hours and keep the tape on until it falls off.

7. Use condoms for the first week.

8. See you in three years unless you decide to remove it sooner.

HOW THE IMPLANT IS REMOVED

1. The nurse or provider will numb the spot with lidocaine, the same as when it was put in.

2. Then she will chat with you for a couple of minutes while the numbing takes effect.

3. Then the nurse will make a tiny incision about an eighth of an inch long over one end of the implant with a scalpel. She will dab the area with gauze if it bleeds, then push on the other side of the implant so the end pokes out of the tiny cut. Then

she will grasp the end and gently pull it out. She will show you
that it is out and intact.

4. She will tape the cut with Steri-Strips, put a square of gauze
    over that, then wrap the whole thing in a stretchy bandage,
    which you will keep on for 24 hours.

Considerations

The implant can stay in for up to three years, but you can have
it removed at any time. I recommend you give it a four- to six-
month trial because any irregular spotting usually stops after
two to three months. But it is up to you, and your provider will
take it out whenever you want.

The IUD—Intrauterine Device

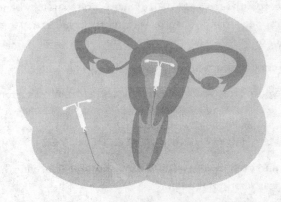

The IUD is a small, T-shaped device that is inserted through the
cervix and into the uterus, where it changes things just enough
to keep sperm from fertilizing your eggs. There are two kinds of
IUDs: hormonal and nonhormonal. I will describe the insertion
process, which is the same for both, after we look at the advantages and disadvantages of the two types separately.

Progestin-Containing IUDs

The Mirena, Skyla, Kyleena, and Liletta IUDs contain a small amount of a slow-release progestin that prevents ovulation and thickens the cervical mucus. With the IUD, the hormone is released right where it is needed, so it takes much smaller amounts to be effective and therefore has fewer side effects than other progestin-only methods.

Progestin IUDs cause almost all their users' periods to lighten and disappear while the IUD is in. These IUDs last between three and eight years. Among the several different brands available, the Skyla is slightly smaller and was designed to market to teens with still-growing bodies. In exchange for being a few millimeters smaller than the others, it lasts for only three years, and women tend to still have light monthly periods with it. The Mirena, Kyleena, and Liletta are all the same size, last for five to eight years, and teens can choose to use those as well. There is no age minimum for any IUD.

Effectiveness

In real-life use: over 99 percent effective. Highly effective!

Advantages

* The progestin in hormone-containing IUDs causes about 80 percent of users to have light or absent periods for years while the IUD is in. In fact, the Mirena IUD is FDA approved to treat heavy, painful periods.
* The IUD is easy to use—once it is in there is nothing to do— and *it's party-ready*.
* Eight years of protection from pregnancy in exchange for a 10-minute office procedure is a pretty awesome deal.
* No one can see that you have it.

* Once it is in, you don't feel it.
* It's safe for smokers and women with medical conditions that make the pill or other estrogen-containing methods risky to use.
* Many women experience no side effects other than very light or absent periods.
* The IUD can be put in as part of abortion care right after the procedure. It can also be put in immediately after giving birth. And it can be used as emergency contraception if put in within five days of unprotected sex. *It is the only method of emergency contraception that then goes on to provide up to 12 years of highly effective birth control.*

Disadvantages

* Most progestin IUD users experience spotting and irregular bleeding for up to three months after insertion, before the periods disappear. On average, women may experience up to 10 days a month of spotting during the initial three months. If you hang in there, it stops after three months in almost all cases, but it can be annoying!
* Some people experience moodiness, weight changes, acne, and other side effects. They are rare, but they do happen.
* For some women, the insertion process is an intense and uncomfortable experience.
* Problems and pregnancy are *extremely* rare (like, one in tens of thousands) but can happen. The IUD can embed in the uterine wall, migrate outside the uterus, or slide out of you all on its own. If a woman does get pregnant with an IUD in place, there is a higher risk of ectopic, or tubal, pregnancy and miscarriage if she wants to continue the pregnancy.

Paragard—The Copper IUD

The nonhormonal IUD used in the United States is called Paragard, and it is the only long-acting, nonhormonal method available. The Paragard IUD has bio-safe copper wrapped around it, which causes subtle chemical changes in the uterine lining that confuse and confound the sperm, making them unable to reach your eggs. You still ovulate and have a monthly period with the Paragard IUD in place. After insertion, your period may be heavier and crampier, especially for the first three to six months. The Paragard can stay in for up to 12 years, making it the birth control method that lasts the longest.

Effectiveness

In real-life use: over 99 percent effective, so *highly effective.*

Advantages

* This method, which takes less than 10 minutes to put in, gives you up to 12 years of more than 99 percent effective birth control with *no hormones.* I mean . . . *boom!*
* No one can see that you have it.
* Once it is in, you don't feel it.
* It's safe for smokers and women with medical conditions that make the pill or other estrogen-containing methods risky to use.
* It can be used as emergency contraception when put in within five days of unprotected sex.
* It can be put in immediately following an abortion or giving birth.

Disadvantages

* Some women find IUD insertion to be intense and uncomfortable.
* The Paragard IUD has one major downside: It makes the period crampier and heavier, especially for the first three to six months after insertion. After a year of use, most women feel their period is only a little bit heavier than it was without the IUD. The period returns to normal after IUD removal. If your period is already heavy and crampy, you may not be very happy with the Paragard IUD. It is an ideal option for people whose periods are generally light and "easy to manage."
* Problems and pregnancy are both extremely rare but can happen. The IUD can embed in the uterine wall, migrate outside the uterus, or slide out of you all on its own. If a woman does get pregnant with an IUD in place, there is a higher risk of ectopic, or tubal, pregnancy and miscarriage if she wants to continue the pregnancy.

HOW THE IUD GOES IN

The IUD insertion procedure takes less than 10 minutes. During those minutes, you have a speculum inside your vagina so your cervix can be seen. The speculum shouldn't hurt, but it feels like a weird sort of pressure. The IUD comes in a very thin tube, which is carefully admitted through the opening of the cervix (the os) and into your uterus. Then the tube slides back out, but the IUD remains inside. Thin, short strings are left in the cervical os but can only be felt way up inside your vagina. These can be used to check that your IUD is in place and will be used to remove the IUD later.

Before the insertion appointment, make sure you do not have

any unprotected sex for two weeks. If there is any chance you are already pregnant, you cannot have an IUD inserted. If you have had unprotected sex in the past five days, it *can* be put in and will act as emergency contraception for you.

These are ways to make the IUD insertion experience as comfortable as possible:

1. The day of the appointment, eat a good breakfast so you don't get nauseous or dizzy.

2. Take 600 mg of ibuprofen (that is three OTC Motrin pills all at once) with food about an hour before the appointment. This will decrease cramping.

3. If you can get your IUD inserted while you are on your period, it may be easier. I know that sounds odd, but listen—while on your period, your cervix is a little bit open to let the blood out. This makes it easier to slide the insertion tube through.

4. Do your best to take slow, deep breaths and keep your body relaxed during the insertion, which will actually make the insertion more comfortable.

5. Attitude is everything—I see teenagers get IUDs all the time and do very well with the insertion. If you really want it, you *can* do it. Also, be sure you feel good about your provider, who should talk to you, make eye contact with you, and put effort into helping you feel at ease. If they are too busy to do that, then hold off and try getting one elsewhere.

6. Female providers tend to be very gentle and kind when doing IUD insertions because they can relate to what their client is experiencing. I recommend seeking a female provider for your insertion.

These are the insertion steps, which usually include *three period-like cramps*.

1. You will be guided to slide down to the edge of the exam table so your bottom is right at the table's edge, and you will

place your feet in footrests. You will need to drop your knees apart, and the provider will sit on a stool between your legs. A drape will cover your lower body. *Your provider will wear gloves at all times and will never touch you with bare hands*. She will talk you through the entire process, telling you what she is about to do each step of the way, and you can ask her to stop at any time. *It's your body*.

2. The provider will slide a speculum into your vagina and open it just enough to see your cervix. She will adjust her light so she can see your cervix well.

3. Then she will clean your cervix with antiseptic on a big cotton swab, and some may offer to put numbing medicine into your cervix as well, although it is not required.

4. She will grasp your cervix with an instrument that holds it steady while the IUD goes in. You may feel the first cramp with that.

5. She will slide a very thin, sterile rod called a sound through your cervix into your uterus and then right back out again. The sound measures the inside of your uterus so the IUD can be placed exactly where it needs to go. This is the second cramp.

6. Then she will set up the IUD inserter tube to the correct measurement and slide it through your cervix into your uterus. She will adjust it so the arms of the IUD open up when the IUD reaches the top portion of the uterus, count to 10 while the IUD arms fully open, and slide the insertion tube back out. This is the third cramp. Your IUD is in! You are doing amazing!

7. Now she will trim the IUD strings so they are about two or three centimeters long, then remove the cervix-holder and the speculum. Everything is out of you now except your IUD.

8. You will slide back up the table so you are lying on it comfortably and chill there for a few minutes. You may have cramping

during this time, similar to a bad period, but it usually fades within a few minutes. If you feel dizzy or weird, your clinic staff can bring you water or a cool compress, or run a fan.

9. While most women walk out after an IUD insertion feeling fine, some women feel crampy for the rest of the day. If this is you, go home, rest, and keep taking ibuprofen every four to six hours. The aftercare instructions are no tub baths or swimming for two days and no sex for a week while your body gets used to it, and then you are good to go! A follow-up appointment is made for four weeks out.

HOW TO CHECK YOUR IUD

After the IUD has been in for three weeks or so, you can check for your strings. Squat on the floor, lay on your bed with your legs open, or stand with one foot up on the toilet. Slide a clean finger into your vagina and sweep around in the very back. Your cervix feels like a nose way up in there. You should be able to feel the fishing-line-like IUD strings on your cervix. You can check your strings any time you're wondering if your IUD is in place or not. If it is in place, it is working. If you cannot find the strings, use condoms until you can come in and be checked. Some women check their strings regularly and some never do. We recommend checking once a year if you think of it.

HOW THE IUD IS REMOVED

The good news is that removal is easy! The hard part was getting it in, and that is already done. You *will* have to get on the table with your bottom on the edge and your feet in footrests again. The nurse will slide in a speculum, grasp the strings with a tool called a ring forceps, and gently pull until the IUD comes out through the cervix. The bendy arms of the T bend up as it comes through. The removal takes only a few seconds and doesn't really hurt.

You can have your IUD removed anytime you want.

Considerations

Some women come back after insertion and say their partner can feel the IUD poking them. It is not the IUD they are feeling, it's *the strings*. If your partner is complaining, squat on the floor and, with a clean finger, feel for your strings. When you feel them, try to sweep them to the side so they wrap around the cervix to one side. Then the ends won't be pointing down. They usually soften and do this on their own after a few weeks.

Rumor: IUDs work by causing little abortions every month.

Fact: Both types of IUDs work by preventing conception. *IUDs are not abortifacients*. The progestin IUDs prevent ovulation and thicken the cervical mucus so the sperm cannot enter the uterus. The copper in the Paragard decreases sperm mobility so the sperm cannot reach your eggs. In both cases, there is no conception, so there is nothing to abort. This rumor harms women by scaring them with untruths and thereby limiting their choices.

Honorable Mention: Sterilization

There is one more birth control method available, but it's not for teenagers or young adults. I am still going to mention it so you know about it. Sterilization is a surgical procedure that results in a permanent end to a person's fertility. A woman is sterilized by tubal ligation, a surgery in which the fallopian tubes are cut and tied so sperm can never again reach her eggs. For a man, the procedure is a vasectomy, where the tube containing sperm is cut and tied. For both men and women, sterilization is considered permanent and irreversible. While there are procedures that can be done to reverse vasectomies, they are not guaranteed to work. A pregnancy is about 50 percent likely after a vasectomy reversal. A teenager cannot consent to sterilization, nor can an adult consent on a teenager's behalf. In the United States, it is virtually impossible to convince a doctor to sterilize someone under 35 because people *do* change their minds about wanting children. But know, down the road of your life, it may be something you choose to do later.

STORIES FROM THE CLINIC

Asher was a 21-year-old nonbinary person with a uterus. They had a male-bodied partner and used Nexplanon for birth control. They were considering starting female-to-male gender-affirming hormone therapy at some point in the next few years. In the meantime, Asher liked the fact that the Nexplanon gave them both effective contraception and no periods.

Cassidy was a young teenager when she had an appointment with me in the clinic and announced that she had come in for a Skyla IUD. At first I wanted to talk her out of it because she was young and had only had sex twice. But Cassidy stated she would only be comfortable having sex again if she had the level of protection that an IUD provides. She had done her research, knew what the insertion procedure involved, and felt she could handle it. There is no medical age minimum for an IUD, and I realized if she wanted it, she should have it. We went over her medical history, and then I inserted her IUD for her. The insertion went smooth as butter. The cramps she experienced were very mild, and she walked out of the clinic feeling great. At her one-month follow-up visit she told me she was very happy with her IUD, and was relieved she did not have to think about birth control again until she turned 17.

Jesalyn came in for a Mirena IUD insertion. When I went to insert the speculum into her vagina, she got very anxious and clenched her muscles tight. I tried to help her relax, but she was very uncomfortable with the exam. I stopped what I was doing, and we talked about her options again. She decided to try the Nexplanon instead. She handled the Nexplanon insertion like a boss and left the clinic satisfied that she still got long-acting birth control, even if it wasn't the IUD after all.

Journal Prompt/Reflections

* Describe your thoughts about long-acting birth control.
* What might be some advantages of it for you? What might be the disadvantages?
* Was any of the information in this chapter new or surprising? How so?

7

Sexually Transmitted Infections

A Story from the Clinic

When I opened the door and walked into the exam room, the young woman sitting on the table burst into tears. She was a new college student, away from home for the first time like so many people in our town. On this morning, she could hardly walk due to the pain between her legs and was desperate for help before her final exams next week. I handed her a tissue and she wiped her eyes.

"I'm really mad," she said. "I have been seeing this new guy for a month. He seemed so nice, but he never said *anything* about having an STI and I am pretty sure he has given me some-thing. . . ."

I asked for details about her symptoms, and she said the painful sores around the outside of her vagina came up three days ago. She felt slightly feverish the day before that. The sores were so raw it was hurting her to pee.

"Have you ever had symptoms like these before?" I asked.

She shook her head no.

I pulled the footrests out of the exam table and guided her feet to their soft fleece coverings. I gloved up, turned on the

light, and took a look. I swabbed a couple of the sores with a special cotton swab to run a viral culture. Then I helped her sit up.

"Take a deep breath," I said. "I will tell you what I see."

I had to give her some hard news.

"It looks like you are having a herpes outbreak," I said. "We
cannot be 100 percent certain until the culture comes back in
four or five days. I want to treat you today anyway so you can
start feeling better. Because you have never had it before, this
is your primary outbreak. The good news is, it is the most painful outbreak you will ever have. Because it is new to you, your
body doesn't recognize it. Now your body will start to build
up immunity to the virus, and future outbreaks will be less
severe."

"Now that I have it, I will always have it?" she asked.

"Yes," I said. "But please understand, it does not impact
your health beyond occasional outbreaks. And, it is so common that perhaps 30 percent of the population in the United
States has it."

I gave her handouts and counseled her about hygiene; boost-
ing her immune system with stress management, extra sleep,
and good nutrition; and how to protect sexual partners from contracting it. Her future sex partners would need to be informed
that she had this. She left with a bag of 36 condoms and a prescription for acyclovir, which would clear up the sores within a
few days. She would feel better in time to take her finals.

She came back in a week for follow-up and the test results.
The test came back positive for herpes simplex virus. The acyclovir had worked, and the sores were almost gone. She felt
well enough to study over the weekend and was set to take her
finals. She was still upset about having herpes, but life would
go on.

The Deal with STIs

The term "STI" stands for sexually transmitted infections, meaning they are infections that are spread through sexual contact. STIs can be spread through all kinds of sex, not just penis-in-vagina sex. Oral sex, anal sex, queer sex, and sex toys can all put you at varying risk of STIs. We don't call them STDs anymore because that stood for sexually transmitted diseases, which made it sound like people who had them were diseased and something was wrong with *them*.

STIs are common. Common colds get passed around, and so do STIs. You can get one from your first partner or your 14th. In the United States, between 10 million and 12 million people between 18 and 24 get STIs a year. Up to one in four sexually active teen women have an STI at any time.

People often feel "bad" or "dirty" if they are diagnosed with an STI. It's time to drop the shame factor. As I mentioned above, STIs are extremely common, so if you get one, there is no point in blaming yourself or feeling bad about yourself. When we drop the stigma around STIs we make it easier for people to share information with partners and to get testing and treatment. STIs don't define who you are as a person, but they *do* need to be treated.

Let's take a look at the most common STIs.

Chlamydia: The most common STI among people under 24, chlamydia is a bacterial infection that primarily affects the cervix, bladder, and uterus in women. Most common symptoms in females are green, foul-smelling discharge; pelvic pain; pain with sex; and pain with urination.

In men, it causes burning with urination and a penile discharge or "drip." Both men and women can have it for months without symptoms.

People can also get chlamydia infections in the throat from oral sex or in the rectum from anal sex.

It can take two weeks after exposure to chlamydia before you test positive. This is called the incubation period—the time it takes for an infection to develop after exposure to it. (Different kinds of infections have different incubation periods.) You will test negative for something in the window between exposure and infection development.

If untreated, chlamydia can climb into the uterus and ovaries, causing pelvic inflammatory disease (PID). This is a very serious and painful infection that can scar the fallopian tubes and contribute to infertility.

It is completely curable with antibiotics.

You only need to have unprotected sex *one time* with someone who has it to catch it.

You should retest two months after treatment to be sure it is gone. That is called taking a test of cure.

Gonorrhea: A bacterial infection with similar symptoms to chlamydia, gonorrhea can also lead to PID. It is not as common as chlamydia.

Green discharge, bad odor, pain with sex, and pelvic pain are the most common symptoms women have. This infection can also colonize the throat, causing a sore throat, or the anus.

Gonorrhea is completely curable with an injection of antibiotics.

You can have both chlamydia and gonorrhea at once. You only need to have sex once with someone to catch it.

You should retest two months after treatment to be sure it is gone.

Trichomoniasis (Trich): This infection lives primarily in the vagina, where it causes profuse runny, smelly, green or yellow vaginal discharge and redness/irritation of the vagina and vulva.

Men can pass it around without having symptoms, so both partners need treatment if a woman has it.

Trich is completely curable with an antibiotic called metronidazole, or Flagyl, although sometimes it is treatment resistant and takes a few rounds with different medicines.

It used to be diagnosed with a pelvic exam to obtain a microscope slide of your discharge, but now there is a urine test for it, so you can just pee in a cup. Progress!

You should have a retest a month after treatment to be sure it is gone.

Genital Warts: These are fleshy warts that appear on the vulva, bikini area, vaginal opening, anus, inner thighs, or buttocks. They develop lobes, giving them a "cauliflower" appearance. They are caused by infection with human papilloma virus (HPV).

They can be frozen or burned off at a clinic but might pop up again until your body clears out the virus that causes them.

HPV is extremely common. It gets passed around and then cleared out of bodies with such frequency that most people don't know they have it unless they develop warts. The virus can also cause cervical cancer in women over 21, which is what the Pap smear screens for.

Because warts can be on body parts not covered by a condom, condoms don't protect you fully against HPV/genital warts. Better to look closely at someone to check for warts before you engage in sex with them.

The good news is that HPV comes and goes, and your immune

system can clear it completely from your body within about two years of infection. So your body will cure itself of HPV infection over time, but then you can catch it again.

If you are over 21, a Pap smear every three years screens you for cellular changes associated with cervical cancer.

Herpes: Herpes is caused by two varieties of the herpes simplex virus (HSV): HSV 1 and HSV 2. Somewhere between 10 percent and 30 percent of the American population tests positive for the herpes virus. That means if you walk into a room with 10 people, between one and three of them have herpes or are carriers of it. It is *common* in the population.

We used to call HSV 1 "oral herpes" because in the past it was the strain responsible for cold sores on the mouth. However, nowadays there has been so much cross-infection between genitals and mouths, that is not true anymore.

Herpes is not curable, but it is manageable. It lives dormant in a person's sacral spinal nerves between outbreaks.

The initial outbreak is always the most intense and painful because your immune system doesn't recognize it. There can be prodromal symptoms for a couple of days before sores appear. These symptoms might include a low-grade fever, tingling sensations in the genital area, or sacral nerve pain. Over the years following initial infection, the outbreaks occur less frequently, and there are lifestyle changes you can make to support your immune system function.

If you have ever had an outbreak, you can spread it to someone else, so you need to tell potential sex partners that you have it. Then they can decide what level of risk they are willing to take. People with herpes go on to lead normal lives with sex and love and babies and all the things. It might feel like the end of the world at first, but it is not.

Once exposed, you will always test positive as a carrier, regardless of whether you have ever had an outbreak or a cold sore. Once you have tested positive, you never need to be tested again.

The sores themselves are extremely contagious, so avoid touching anyone's *anything* if you notice an open blister or sore on their mouth, genitals, thigh, buttocks, or vulva. Even sharing drinks can spread it if the sore is on their mouth.

Condoms do not necessarily cover the sores, so they aren't fully protective against herpes. They do protect against some of the viral shedding but not all. A visual check of your partner and an honest, thorough conversation about herpes histories can help make herpes infection less likely.

A viral culture is positive right away but takes five to seven days for results. The blood test for antibodies takes several weeks after exposure before it turns positive.

Cold sores: Some people have gotten cold sores since childhood. They may only rarely get them, such as when they have been sick and their immune system is low. You do not need to entirely avoid sex with someone who has a history of cold sores, but you should avoid contact with them if they currently have a sore.

Cross contamination from mouth to genitals: If a partner has a cold sore on their mouth and they give you oral sex, you can get sores on your genitals.

Molluscum contagiosum: These small, painless round bumps can pop up on the genitals, vulva, thighs, lower belly, and buttocks after exposure to someone who has them. You can also get them from sheets, towels, and bedding. Sometimes they get spread at waxing studios. The bumps get a pearly white head but are hard to pop without using a needle. They will eventually go away on their own, but it can take years. A provider at a clinic can freeze them or scrape them for you, speeding their disappearance.

Syphilis: Syphilis is a very serious STI because, if left untreated, it can cause blindness, insanity, and eventually death.

Syphilis was extremely rare for many years but is seeing a comeback these days. During the COVID pandemic, we called it "the other pandemic" at my clinic because we saw *so many cases of it*.

The progression of syphilis takes years. It starts with a single, mostly painless sore called a chancre at the point of infection, usually on the genitals, which goes away on its own. After several months, a rash on the hands, feet, or chest appears and then goes away. Then there can be a latent period of many years—if left untreated, the disease eventually climbs into a person's neurological system, causing blindness, madness, and then death.

In many cases, the first couple of symptoms (i.e., the sore and the rash) are missed as symptoms worth investigating. Some people are prone to rashes and sores, and they don't worry much about them. This is why it is common for syphilis to be first detected only by blood test. And that is why it is so important to get tested regularly.

Test results aren't positive until four to six weeks after exposure. If there is any question, retest!

Syphilis is completely curable with injectable penicillin. You will need either one shot or a series of three over the course of a few weeks depending on which stage of infection you are in. Further blood tests can help determine which stage of the disease it is.

If you are diagnosed with syphilis, you will need blood tests after treatment every three to four months for a year to be sure it is gone-daddy-gone and not just hiding.

HIV: Human immunodeficiency virus is a sexually transmitted virus that attacks your immune system, leading to serious illness by any number of opportunistic infections.

In the 1980s, when this STI first appeared on the scene, over 100,000 people died from it. Nowadays, thanks to advances in modern medicine, medication regimens keep people with HIV alive for normal life spans. You still don't want to get it.

There is no cure—it is a lifer.

Condoms and dental dams are extremely effective at protecting you against HIV, especially when used with all the types of sex: oral, anal, and penis in vagina.

Test results aren't positive until four to six weeks after exposure.

How to Protect Yourself from STIs

The official definition of "safe sex" is sexual activity that does not involve exchange of body fluids, including semen, vaginal fluids, and blood. But the way I approach it is that protecting yourself from STIs requires a three-pronged approach:

1. Condom/dental dam use
2. STI testing and treatment
3. Communication

Condom Use

Condoms are a barrier that protects against almost all the STIs. Women are particularly susceptible to catching STIs through penis-in-vagina sex because the tissues of the vagina are very porous and absorbent. *Remember, using a water-based lube, such as K-Y or Astroglide, in addition to the lube that comes on the condom increases pleasure for you and decreases irritation.*

Condom Use and Nonmonogamy: For people who engage in hookups, casual sex, concurrent partners, polyamory, or any form of nonmonogamy, I recommend you consider condoms essential players in your game. Just because a guy likes you enough to have sex with you does not mean he is taking care of your health and safety. *You have to do that.*

If you are hooking up and he tells you he doesn't like to use condoms, and you choose to go ahead anyway, during that sex you will be exposed to bacteria and viruses from *everyone else* he has slept with. If he is not using condoms with you, he has not used condoms with the girl last weekend or the one from the week before. And so on. Not only do condoms protect you from STIs, but they leave your body cleaner too. After sex, his ejaculate and fluids come out neatly in the condom.

Note: Some people enjoy "fluid bonding" with their partners, sharing body fluids as a way of deepening connection and intimacy. Everything is your own choice to make, but I recommend you consider the risks and benefits before deciding. Fluid bonding can be navigated to minimize risks, but it takes commitment to consent and communication from all parties involved.

When You Want to Use Condoms and He Does Not: It is hard to handle pressure by a sex partner trying to get you to do things you don't really want to do, including having sex without a condom. (We will explore more about consent and boundaries in chapter 10.) Girls are generally raised to please others. Our whole culture constantly puts out subtle messages, telling girls that being pleasant and pleasing others is what we are supposed to do. On top of that, we have this intense need to be liked, and we are excited to be *desired* by males we find attractive.

But remember, *you* possess something of value in the

dynamic with him—your precious body, your vagina. So own your value and leverage your power. Share your body in sexual intimacy if you want to, but do it in a way that is safe and feels right for you. What's the worst thing that could happen if you insist on condoms? He would change his mind about having sex, and then you would feel disappointed? Maybe he will learn not to expect sex without condoms. As poet and author Maya Angelou says, "Each time a woman stands up for herself . . . she stands up for all women."

Condom Use and Monogamy: When people have one steady sex partner or boyfriend, I recommend they use condoms at the beginning of the relationship and both get STI tested. Once six weeks have passed since either of you have had sex with other people, you both get negative STI testing results, and there is a commitment to ongoing monogamy, the condom use can discontinue.

Condom Use and Current STI: If you and your partner are both being treated for an STI, you need to avoid sex for a week after treatment, then use condoms for a week after that. Otherwise you will likely reinfect each other and have to be treated all over again.

Rumor: I have a boyfriend, so I don't have to use condoms with him, right?

Fact: Many women ask this in my clinic. I usually answer by asking *them* a question in return: "Are you sure he is not sleeping with anybody else?"

If my clients look away and say things like, "Uh, I don't know what he does when he is not with me" or "I'm not sure, I don't *think* so. . . . " then the answer is, *you still need to use condoms.*

You cannot assume a sex partner is monogamous with you just because you are "seeing each other." It is very common for people to have concurrent partners and to be nonmonogamous.

Unfortunately, some partners are not honest about it either. Often, you can probably tell. When a partner is committed to monogamy with you, you can usually *feel* it in your gut. You *know* where he is when you are not together. You have that level of close connection. If there is any doubt, protect yourself. *When your sex partner and you agree to be monogamous and have both been STI tested with negative results at least six weeks since either of you have had sex with anyone else, you may choose to have sex without condoms.* In any situation less certain than that, it is always going to be a risk.

STI Testing and Treatment

If you are a sexually active person under 25, I recommend getting STI tested every three to six months. Any time you change partners, have a hookup or a casual partner, or experience nonconsensual sex, you should get tested. If your lifestyle involves more than one partner, testing routinely every three to four months will make sure that, if you do have something, you can treat it before it develops into a more serious infection, which will keep you from becoming part of the dreaded spread.

Testing for gonorrhea, chlamydia, and trichomoniasis is easy—you go to a clinic like Planned Parenthood, a college health center, or your county health department and pee in a cup. To find a place for STI testing, go to gettested.cdc.gov and enter the ZIP code where you are. Test results usually come in three to five days. HIV and syphilis are tested by a blood draw. "STI testing" routinely consists of testing for these five STIs.

The antibodies to herpes can also be tested by blood, which tells you if you have been exposed but not if you have active disease. For that, you need to have a viral culture done if/when you develop symptoms. The throat and anus can also be swabbed for chlamydia and gonorrhea. The only test for HPV is the Pap smear, which you will get when you are 21. If you think you might have genital warts or molluscum, you can go to a clinic or the health department to be checked and get them removed.

Communication

Clear communication with prospective sex partners and ongoing check-ins with current partners are tools in your STI prevention kit. If you don't ask, then you may not find out until it is too late.

Yeah, it is awkward to discuss STIs in the heat of the moment. You are really into a guy, he is finally alone with you . . . and you are gonna ask about his STI history? Yup. Trust me, it is even more awkward to have to call people you have had sex with to tell them you have an STI and may have given it to them. Cure is cool, but prevention is better.

Before having sex, discuss the following:

* When was the last time you were STI tested?
* Was anything positive?
* Were you treated, and did you go back to get a negative result after?
* How many partners have you had in the past four months?
* Do you currently have other partners? Do you use condoms with them?
* Have you ever had sores, warts, or herpes breakouts?
* Do you get cold sores? When was the last time you had one?

People can be manipulative and dishonest, unfortunately. But you increase your chances of sensing the truth if you bring up the topic in a straightforward manner and watch for nonverbal cues for honesty. Watch them as they talk. Is your partner looking into your eyes or looking away? Are they mumbling and stuttering, saying something and then backtracking, or talking clearly? Do they know what they had, what they took for it? Are they being vague or specific? Because there is no vague STI. These things are all clues about honesty and awareness of sexual health.

HOW TO TELL A PARTNER YOU TESTED POSITIVE FOR AN STI

* Think about what you want to say. You can even practice if you are nervous. Remember, you are doing the right thing.

* Make space for the conversation to take place in a calm, private environment.

* Give the information in clear language. Be prepared to calmly listen to your partner's initial reaction, which may be emotional. Try not to get defensive or take it personally.

* Offer resources for next steps: where your partner can go to get tested and treated as well. Some clinics send patients home with treatments for themselves and their partners.

* *Remember, you should refrain from having sex until both of you have completed treatment and waited one additional week post-treatment to prevent reinfection.*

SAFE NON-PENIS-IN-VAGINA AND QUEER SEX

I'm going to take this moment to explore how to be safe with types of sex other than penis-in-vagina sex. Touch or sexual contact of any kind requires consideration of boundaries and full consent. Chapter 10 delves deeply into agency, boundaries, and consent, and all of it applies here. The kinds of sex in this section can happen between two people with vaginas; two people with penises; more than two people; or any combination of people, including one person with a penis and one with a vagina. We will start with sexual touch least risky for STI exposure (the least possibility for exchange of body fluids) and move up to the sex with highest risk of STI exposure.

1. Dry humping, grinding. Rubbing your body against someone else while clothed or partially clothed is a pleasurable way to touch and connect that has no risk of STI because there is no exchange of body fluids.

2. Touch of skin, massage of back, legs, arms (the skin of the inner arm is very sensitive), backs of knees, neck, etc. All of this is sensual and pleasurable, with no risk of STI.

3. Hand play. Includes chest and nipple stimulation, touch and stimulation of external genitalia, and penetrative fingering. Hand play can be a vector of STI if the same hand touches two people's genitals and body fluids. To minimize risk, wash hands before play, trim fingernails, and use gloves with lube for extra protection. Never go from anal to vaginal fingering without washing hands or changing gloves. Two people with vaginas can pass the bacteria that cause bacterial vaginosis and trich through hand play, so use the precautions above to prevent that.

4. Toys. Vibrators, dildos, anal beads, and strap-on dildos are common additions to queer sex. Toys can be a vector for STIs if they have one person's body fluids on them and then are

inserted into another person's body. To be safe, wash and disinfect toys between use and between people. You can use condoms on anything that is inserted into a body part; just be sure to add plenty of water-based lube. Change the condoms between people if the toy will be shared. For specialized sex toy disinfectant, go to www.goodvibes.com.

5. Oral sex, mouth to vulva/clit/vagina. Many people with vaginas find mouth to genitalia sex to be one of the most pleasurable forms of sexual touch. However, there is a risk of STIs. The receiver of oral sex can get herpes on their genitals from an infected mouth, so always check that your partner does not have any mouth sores before consenting to receiving oral sex. The giver can get herpes, and it is also possible for HPV and other STIs to be passed into the throat. There is a way to protect both of you: Dental dams are squares of clear, thin plastic wrap–like material that provide barrier protection. You can also cut open a condom and make a square-shaped barrier to lay over the clit/vulva. The risk of HIV to the giver of mouth-to-vulva sex is very low.

6. Oral sex, mouth to penis (blow jobs, giving head). The giver of mouth-to-penis sex can contract chlamydia and gonorrhea in the throat and also can get herpes, HPV, syphilis, and HIV from penile contact. The receiver can get herpes, syphilis, and other STIs from the giver's mouth. Condoms protect both of you against these infections.

7. Mouth to anus sex. This carries risk of all the STIs to both parties. Use a dental dam or cut open a condom and make a square-shaped barrier for safe sex.

8. Anal sex. The recipient of penetrative anal sex is especially vulnerable to STIs because the skin of the anus is easily damaged, and microtears in the skin can lead to blood-borne infections, such as HIV and Hepatitis B and C, as well as all the other STIs. For this reason, condom use is recommended when engaging in anal sex. Tip: Prior to anal pene-

tration, apply a ton of water-based lube to both condom and
anus. The anus does not produce *any* lubrication of its own,
so you need more lube than you would think.

*Remember, one condom or glove per body part. When ready to
switch bodies or body parts, change the condom or glove to a
fresh one.*

Honorable Mentions: The Pap Smear

The Pap smear is a screening test for both cervical cancer and
the presence of HPV in the cervix, which is associated with cervical cancer. We used to do these every year, so we called them
"annual exams." The latest guidelines recommend that people
with uteruses have them every three years. People under 21 do
not need them because, even if they do have HPV, their youth-
ful health protects them from developing anything serious and
their bodies/immune systems will clear it out on their own.

The Pap smear is obtained during a pelvic exam. A person
having one lies on an exam table, legs open, feet in footrests. A
nurse or clinician will insert a speculum to see the cervix and
adjust her light so she can visualize it completely. She then will
brush the cervix with a special brush that collects cells from its
surface. This will not hurt, but there may be a brief odd sensation. The speculum will be removed and the cells obtained are
prepped for the lab, where they will be tested for abnormalities
and the presence of HPV infection. If there are abnormal cells
or HPV infection, a plan for further testing will be made at a
follow-up visit. If results are all normal, another Pap should be
done in three years.

Journal Prompts/Reflections

* Would you describe your sexual lifestyle as abstinence, monogamy, nonmonogamy, or casual hookups? Given your lifestyle, how well are you protecting yourself from STIs? If you are not using condoms and know you are putting yourself at risk, what are the reasons for that? Reflect on what you could do differently.

* Think about sexual politics and power. In this chapter, I stated, "*You* possess something of value [. . .] your vagina. So own your value and leverage your power." What do you think I mean by that statement? Have you ever thought about dynamics between men and women that way? What does it mean for a woman to see her body as something of value, something precious worth standing up for? What are some reasons women don't always value themselves and their bodies? How can we change that?

* This is a repeat prompt from an earlier chapter, but if you did not do it then, here is another chance. Successful condom use requires preplanning. Where are some places you could keep condoms so they would easily be on hand in case you need them? (Okay, this was a trick question. Now put away this book and, if you have condoms already, go put them in those places; if not, go buy some and do it.)

8

The V-Word

Taking Charge of Your Vaginal Health

V-words: vulva and vagina. First off, let's clear up any confusion you might have about the difference between vulvas and vaginas. These words are not interchangeable; they refer to different things. The vulva is the part of your body that is *outside* and around your vagina. The vagina is the tube *inside* you that leads to your cervix, the entrance to your uterus and fallopian tubes.

The vulva includes the clitoris, the inner and outer labia (lips), the perineum (the flesh between your vagina and anus), the introitus (vaginal opening), and the mons pubis (where your pubic hair grows).

The vagina is the part that is actually inside you. It is a tube, about three inches long, but stretchy and full of little folds called rugae. Menstrual blood comes out of the vagina during the period, the baby comes out of it during childbirth, and the penis goes in during intercourse. When a female is sexually aroused, her vagina expands and lubricates itself. It expands enough to lift the cervix and uterus up so they are less likely to be bumped by the penis. That is one of the reasons why sex is more comfortable for a woman when she is fully aroused.

When you get a chance, take a good look at your vulva to become more familiar with it. Get a hand mirror, lie on your bed with your legs open, and then hold the mirror between your legs, tilted so you can see. A flashlight can be used if needed. You may notice your vulva's dampness; its color, either darker or pinker than the rest of you; and that your labia are uneven. One side is almost always bigger than the other, and the inner lips or outer lips may be larger. Your clitoris may be mostly hidden under its hood or protruding out. (Find it at the top of the vagina above the spot where the inner lips meet.) Everyone's vulva looks unique, just like our faces do.

You can give yourself a visual exam like this every once in a while and check for warts, bumps, discharge, or other changes.

Your vagina will look, feel, and smell healthy when several factors of your inner ecosystem are in balance. Inner ecosystem? Yes. Your vagina and vulva are both mucous membranes, similar to your lips and mouth. In fact, *labia* means "lips"—they are your vagina's lips. Because they are mucous membranes, they are different from the rest of your skin and need to be cared for differently. The skin of mucus membranes is very thin and sensitive (like your lips) but makes its own lubrication/wetness that serves as a protective barrier against pathogens. That is why your inner labia, vaginal opening, and vagina are a little damp, wet, or shiny with moisture. That wetness is supposed to be there; it keeps your vagina healthy.

Like your mouth, your vagina is full of "good" bacteria that help to maintain health. Your vaginal flora makes up a microscopic ecosystem, like a garden alive with different herbal plants and flowers. Your vaginal flora maintains the ecosystem's balance and helps fight off infections. The products of its metabolism keeps the pH of the vagina low and acidic, which is good for it. Many things can shift the pH balance, including overcleaning, overheating, and yes, even sex. When things get out of balance, the pH can go up and "bad" bacteria or fungal organisms can overgrow, like invasive weeds in a garden. You may develop a vaginal infection with symptoms like itchiness, irritation, or a discharge. The two most common vaginal infections are yeast infections and bacterial vaginosis (BV). They are both easily treated, and then you can take steps to keep the ecosystem of your vagina in balance.

Principles of Vaginal Health

Hygiene

The vagina is a self-cleaning organ. It does not need to be cleaned with purchased products. Let me repeat that. *The vagina is a self-cleaning organ.* When women first see the word "bacteria," they immediately think, "Oh no, that's bad. I'm going to clean it really well and get rid of it." But remember: Not all bacteria are bad. Our immune and digestive systems rely on good bacteria for optimal functioning. The same goes with our vaginas—we need the right kind of bacteria to maintain vaginal health.

If your vagina has an unusual odor or other symptom, that indicates something is off balance and there may be an infection brewing. Using a douche or any scented product to clean inside will make it worse by flushing out the good bacteria and stripping away your vaginal mucosa's protective moisture barrier, further disrupting its delicate balance. The douche products found in a drugstore tend to do more harm than good. Soaps and cleaners should only be used around the outer lips, anus, mons, and thighs, never on the delicate vulvar tissues. Water is enough to clean those parts. Using scented soaps and cleansers *near* the vagina is enough to cause irritation in some women. The vagina produces its own discharge to clear out irritants, and one should never attempt to wash inside it.

What you *can* do for vaginal hygiene and health:

Always Wipe from Front to Back: This is the most basic and important aspect to vaginal hygiene. Your poop and your anus are full of the kind of bacteria that overthrow your "good" bacteria and grow into infections. If you are having loose stools, you can shower and wash the anal area after pooping for added protection.

Keep It Cool: Keep the area between your legs from getting too hot or too wet for too long. Excess moisture and heat can cause pathogens such as yeast to proliferate and cause infection. For optimal vaginal hygiene and health:

* Wear cotton underwear instead of synthetic because cotton breathes and stays drier, while synthetics trap moisture and heat.
* Change out of sweaty, tight gym clothes after working out. Don't just wear them for the rest of the day.
* Same with wet bathing suits—spending the day in a sopping-wet suit can cause vaginal irritation in some women. So after pool or beach time, change!
* Fashion choice villain #1—*the thong!* Check it out—the little string that sits inside your butt crack? Well, that makes a perfect ladder for bacteria to use to climb from your a-hole into your vagina. Gross, right? If a woman is prone to

vaginal infections, the number one way she can decrease their incidence is by ditching thong underwear. Seriously. Thongs were not designed with your health in mind.

* Fashion choice villain #2—living in tight synthetic (spandex) leggings. Even if you are not working up a sweat, if you wear synthetic leggings all day long, you are probably cooking your vagina. If you are having issues, switch to cotton leggings, skirts, or looser, flowy pants and see if I am right.

Eat Probiotic Foods: Probiotic foods, or "live" foods, add the good kind of bacteria into your system, while stress, alcohol, antibiotic use, and other lifestyle factors diminish them. Probiotic foods support and strengthen your vaginal flora. Lactobacilli are one of the most common types of "good" bacteria found in the vagina. They are also found in "live" foods like yogurt, yogurt drinks and smoothies, kefir, and kombucha. Sauerkraut and pickled foods are rich in lactobacilli. You can buy probiotic supplements, but those might be a waste of money because the bacteria might be dead already before you take them, and there is no way to know. Probiotic pills that have been kept in refrigerators at the store are your best bet. But if you eat live foods, you know you are getting live bacteria.

Wear Condoms: Not this again! But seriously, here is another great reason to bag it. Semen has a very high pH. Some women notice they get a fishy smell or vaginal infection frequently after sex with certain partners. It's the ejaculate, raising the vaginal pH and throwing the delicate ecosystem off. Not only that, but a man's penis can be colonized by the bacteria from other people's vaginas. Because everyone's flora is uniquely *theirs*, when a condomless penis introduces other women's bacteria into your vagina, it can throw your ecosystem off.

Yeast Infections

What It Is: Yeast infections are the most common of the vaginal infections. They are fungal skin infections caused by an organism called *Candida albican*s or sometimes by other strains of candida. Candida is what also causes jock itch in men, and thrush and diaper rash in babies. It is not contagious between partners. Your body has candida as a normal part of your vaginal flora, but it is kept in balance by good bacteria, especially lactobacilli. When something throws the balance off, there can be overgrowth of candida, causing yeast infection symptoms to arise.

What Are the Symptoms: The main symptoms of a yeast infection are a red, itchy, or irritated vagina or vulva. There may be patches of red skin on the vulva, with little red spots outside the borders of the patches, called satellites. These do not blister, but if you itch too much the skin can crack and then scab. Often, there can be a vaginal discharge that is white with chunks like cottage cheese. The discharge is odorless or else has a "yeasty" smell like bread dough. There may be burning and discomfort with sex.

What Causes It: Yeast infections are usually caused by one of two things:

1. Getting your genitals too hot and too wet for too long can make yeast overgrow. As discussed above, some examples of this are wearing tight, sweaty spandex gym clothes all day or spending the day in a wet bathing suit. Synthetic underwear, especially thongs, can lead to yeast infections in someone prone to them. It is not sexually transmitted, but sex may be uncomfortable when you have one.

2. Taking antibiotics causes a die-off of the good bacteria that keep the candida in your vagina in check. It is common to take antibiotics for something unrelated, such as strep throat or a urinary tract infection, and then find yourself with a yeast infection two weeks later.

What Can Be Done: Wear cotton underwear, change out of wet gym clothes, and do what you can to keep yourself cool and dry. Limit or take a break from foods and drinks high in sugar. If you are taking antibiotics, be sure to take probiotics or eat lots of yogurt during treatment and for a few weeks after to replace the good bacteria in your system. You can ask the doctor or provider prescribing the antibiotics for a Diflucan pill as well. Diflucan is a single-dose antifungal medication that treats yeast. It can be taken after a course of antibiotics in a bid to prevent a yeast infection before it starts. Some women put a little plain, unsweetened yogurt on their vulva to soothe it, or insert probiotic capsules (sugar-free only) into their vaginas at bedtime. Make sure anything you put on or in the vagina is sugar-free, as yeast thrives on sugar.

Treatment for yeast infections is available over the counter and can be purchased at any drugstore or pharmacy. The treatments are antifungal creams and suppositories, which go into the vagina at bedtime for one, three, or seven days in a row. The most common medications used for this are miconazole or clotrimazole. I recommend suppositories over cream, as they are less messy and easier to use, and I recommend never doing the one-day version, which doesn't seem to work very well but does cause even more burning and irritation in a lot of people who try it. The three-day treatment works very well. Follow the instructions on the package and insert it right before bed so the medication stays inside and clears away the yeast while you are lying down and sleeping. Symptoms are usually improved after the first night but take five or six days to go away completely. While treating the infection, definitely ditch the thongs, wear cotton, and sleep with no underwear or pants on to let air get there and keep it cool. Avoid sex because it won't feel good and the friction can damage your irritated skin.

If the symptoms do not go away after using over-the-counter treatment, you will need to be seen in a women's health clinic. Or, if it's your first time getting these symptoms, you may want to go in and get checked. The provider will give you a pelvic exam, look at a sample of your discharge under a microscope, and run STI testing. Then she will offer you a prescription for the vaginal treatment, a Diflucan pill, or a combination of both. Once you have been diagnosed at a clinic, you can recognize it if it happens again and get the over-the-counter treatment. And you can play detective to figure it out: Did I take antibiotics for a sinus infection two weeks ago and now this? Did I go in the hot tub and then stay in the wet bathing suit for the rest of the day?

Bacterial Vaginosis

What It Is: BV is caused by an overgrowth of anaerobic, "bad" bacteria in the vagina. It is not sexually transmitted but is sexually associated, meaning some women get BV flare-ups after sex with particular partners, especially after sex without condoms. Sex partners can deliver vaginal flora from their other partners into your vagina. While these are not STIs per se, they can throw off the balance of your flora and result in BV. Non-sex-related things can cause it as well, such as excess wetness and heat in your genitals as discussed in the previous sections of this chapter. Immune system changes from illness or dealing with stress can make you prone to BV. With BV, the vaginal pH becomes higher than normal, so instead of being acidic, the vagina is basic, which allows this kind of infectious bacteria to thrive.

What Are the Symptoms: The hallmark symptom of BV is a fishy smell and a vaginal discharge with a fishy odor. This discharge is usually white and milky. There may be a feeling of vaginal irritation as well as burning/discomfort with sex.

What Can Be Done: Home remedies that bring down the vaginal pH can help decrease BV symptoms and even treat the infections. The most promising of these remedies is boric acid suppositories, which have now been studied in a medical trial that found them effective at treating recurrent BV. Boric acid suppositories designed for vaginal use can be bought at some drugstores and online. They must only be used in the vagina and *never* taken by mouth! (That would poison you.) The suppositories are placed in the vagina at bedtime nightly for one to two weeks or one to two times a week for a couple of months if the BV keeps coming back. But these should not be overused, so please follow the directions on the packaging. A vaginal rinse of one tablespoon of organic apple cider vinegar in a cup of water is an old-time natural remedy for BV.

The medical treatment for BV is antibiotics. You will need to be seen at a clinic or provider's office to obtain the treatment. You will have a pelvic exam (with a microscope slide of the discharge made) as well as STI testing. The antibiotic treatment is either a week of pills twice a day or a vaginal cream used at bedtime for five nights. The pills are a very strong antibiotic called Flagyl, and I do not recommend this as the first choice. These pills cause a die-off of the good bacteria in your digestive tract and your vagina, ultimately weakening your immune system, so they can result in secondary infections and other problems.

It is a better idea to use the cream, which goes into the vagina at bedtime, right where it needs to be. Why disrupt your entire system to target medication to your vagina when you can just use it locally in the first place?

Prevention: Using condoms with sex partners who have other partners can stop the spread of unfriendly bacteria into your vaginal ecosystem. Taking off wet swimsuits, avoiding thongs, and wearing cotton to keep cool—all these same tricks apply. Probiotics put the good bacteria into your body, which naturally lowers your vagina's pH. Avoid douching and using scented products on the genitals. And most important, always wipe from front to back.

Urinary Tract Infections (UTIs)

UTIs are not vaginal infections. They are infections of the bladder and urethra, which happen to be located right in front of the vagina. The symptoms of a UTI can be confused with vaginal symptoms. And a UTI can be caused by sexual intercourse. For all these reasons, I am going to discuss UTIs here.

What It Is: A UTI occurs when bacteria are pushed up into the urethra and then climb into the bladder, where they proliferate and develop into an infection. The most common organisms causing UTIs are *E. coli*, found in poop. UTIs can be caused by a number of things, such as holding your urine too long while traveling or during a rigorous work shift, or wiping back to front. But many women develop UTIs after having sex. The action of thrusting during sex can push bacteria up into the urethra. Somehow this happens more frequently after a lot of sexual activity, so UTIs are sometimes called "the honeymoon sickness."

One trick to prevent UTIs is to make it a habit to always pee after sex. The stream of urine flushes out any bacteria that got pushed in. This means you have to get up to pee before falling asleep. But if you are prone to UTIs, it is worth the effort.

Anal contact with anything that then touches the vagina can contribute to UTI development. Never let a partner go from anal sex to vaginal sex. After anal play, it is a good idea to wash off penis, hands, and fingers before moving to vaginal sex. Condom use during anal sex helps decrease the spread of bacteria as well. Make sure the condom used for anal sex gets taken off and tossed out right away. Remember, you cannot *see* bacteria with your naked eye, but it can still be there and cause an infection.

What Are the Symptoms: The symptoms of a UTI are pain with urination; pelvic pressure; frequency, which means running to the bathroom much more often than usual; and urgency, which is feeling like you cannot hold it. Sometimes it feels like you cannot fully empty your bladder as well.

Low back pain, flank pain on one side or the other, fever, and nausea are all signs that the UTI could be climbing into a kidney, which can result in a much more serious infection requiring IV antibiotics to treat. If you experience these symptoms after battling a UTI, you need to go to an ER or urgent care clinic right away.

What to Do: Drink as much water as you possibly can. Fluids will help to flush out the infection. Avoid drinking alcohol and eating sugar. Cranberry pills and a supplement called D-mannose may help. Unsweetened cranberry juice will acidify the urine and help clear out a UTI, but most cranberry juices are sweetened and will not help at all. You would have to read the label carefully to find one with no sugar added, and it will taste *very* tart. An OTC product called AZO helps relieve the pain with urination but doesn't get rid of the infection.

Sometimes the UTI can be cleared up by drinking a lot of water and taking cranberry. But many women need to go to a clinic to get antibiotics. At a clinic or provider's office, you will pee in a cup and your sample will be analyzed. Usually the UTI can be diagnosed right away, but sometimes further testing is required, in which case your sample will be sent to a lab. If diagnosed with a UTI, you will likely be given a three- to five-day course of antibiotics.

You should feel better after 24 hours on the medication, but make sure you finish the whole course so the infection does not come right back. Occasionally women can have recurrent UTIs, which means getting more than five or six in a year. In these cases, working closely with a provider and taking all the lifestyle precautions and suggestions seriously can resolve them.

9

Understanding Female Sexual Pleasure

First, a story: A college student, let's call her Beth, was attracted to a young man she met in art history class. After hanging out together a few times, he invited her back to his place, and she knew they would hook up. Beth had a couple of boyfriends in high school with whom she had intercourse, but it had never felt great for her. While she enjoyed kissing and making out with them, the intercourse itself didn't really do it for her. Now that she was in college, she hoped that sex with this smart, self-confident guy would be different and she would finally experience an orgasm.

But when they got together, their intimacy fell into a familiar pattern. He was very excited and moved quickly from a few minutes of kissing and massaging her breasts to taking off her clothes, stroking her vulva a few times, and then entering her for sex. The whole thing happened too fast for her to get fully aroused, so she was not as wet as she should be, and it felt like he was hitting something inside. She wanted to be seen as "hot" and "good in bed," so she moaned and wrapped her legs around him anyway. The sex got harder and more aggressive, so she shook to give the impression that she came, and then he ejaculated and finished.

Afterward, he was relaxed and drained of energy, and drifted off to sleep. She lay awake beside him, feeling keyed up and full of conflicting feelings. She wondered if something was wrong with her and if she would ever truly enjoy sex. They got together several more times. She wanted to talk to him about slowing it down and focusing on getting her really turned on first, but she could not bring herself to do it. He thought he knew what she liked already, so when they had sex it was fast and hard like the first time, and she found herself acting like she liked it. She eventually stopped seeing him and came to the clinic to see if something was wrong with her.

There was nothing wrong with Beth at all. She just needed to understand her body's sexual response better. We talked about female arousal and the vital role of foreplay. When a woman is aroused, physical changes take place that make sex feel better for her. Beth knew that arousal caused wetness from her body's own lubrication, but she did not know that arousal also makes the vagina stretch and lengthen, which lifts the uterus and cervix up and out of the way of the penis.

We also discussed the anatomy of the clitoris and its role as the central organ of female sexual pleasure. Beth had unrealistic expectations that her young male partner would know more about female bodies than she did. After the visit, she decided to explore herself through masturbation and experienced her first orgasms alone while gently stroking her clitoris. Once she understood how her body responded to different kinds of touch, she felt comfortable telling sex partners what she liked. She discovered that men really liked this self-confident, less passive version of her evolving self. She didn't always reach orgasm every time she had sex with a man, but it happened often enough, and she always made sure that, at the very least, sex was enjoyable and never hurt.

Tips for Empowered Sex

Female Sexual Pleasure Is a Function of Body, Mind, and Emotions

All three components must be there for most women to feel that sex is *good*. People with male and female bodies tend to have different sexual responses, and our culture mainly focuses on male sex, leaving many women out in the cold when it comes to understanding their sexual pleasure.

Most men are visually stimulated and easily aroused by the sight of a body they find attractive, be this an image, a video, or a living person. Blood rushes to their genitals, engorging the penis, which gets hard and erect. Then, rubbing and stimulation of the penis leads to ejaculation and orgasm. Afterward, the penis softens and the man experiences pleasure and relaxation. The whole trajectory is often linear: It builds in intensity until the climax, and then it is done.

For women, on the other hand, arousal is a process usually involving several factors. Yes, the sight of an attractive partner can turn her on, but there has to be other components as well. Safety and comfort are big ones. Women need to feel safe and comfortable to become aroused. And they need *foreplay*. For example, arousal can be brought on by sensuous touch of erogenous zones, such as ears, neck, breasts, and inner arms and thighs. But it can also arise from flirting and the buildup of desire and intrigue, which are more mental than physical. An intimate dinner, exchanging shoulder rubs in a candle-lit room, even sending romantic texts throughout the day are forms of foreplay. It takes time and exploration for a woman to experience the full range of her sexual pleasure, and sexual enjoyment can be seen as something that develops over time through experimentation and increasing awareness.

Women often have this fantasy that if a guy is good-looking and sexy enough, he will awaken her sex, unlocking her pleasure as if he has a magic key. And that may happen, sometimes, if all the conditions of body, mind, and emotional arousal are aligned. But what is more likely is that she will have to do the unlocking herself through understanding what arouses her and self-exploration to discover what brings her to orgasm. Then, in her sexual relationships, she can explore all of it further. But it starts with herself.

The Problem with Porn

Most people today have looked at porn, either out of curiosity or habitually. The problem with most pornography is that it depicts the male fantasy of what women enjoy, which in reality isn't accurate. In male-directed porn, foreplay is usually very brief, then quickly leads to intense, aggressive sex acts. Porn actresses are very good at pretending to enjoy it, and female watchers of this kind of porn learn to mimic their signifiers of enjoyment: moaning, gasping, crying out, shaking. Porn often perpetrates misunderstandings about female sexuality, confusing curious young men and women alike.

As one 22-year-old woman said when we were discussing this issue: "For women's pleasure, we have it all wrong. Foreplay is considered something that happens for a few minutes before the main event: penis-in-vagina sex. But really, foreplay should be the main course, and the penis-in-vagina sex should be seen as the dessert after."

Arousal and Orgasm

When a woman is sexually aroused, several changes take place in her body. The tissue of the vagina and clitoris fills with blood. The vagina engorges, lifting up the cervix and uterus. The vagina also becomes very lubricated and wet. A feeling of wetness is common when aroused, along with sensations of tingling and warmth in the pelvis and a pleasurable pressure in the clitoris.

Clitoris

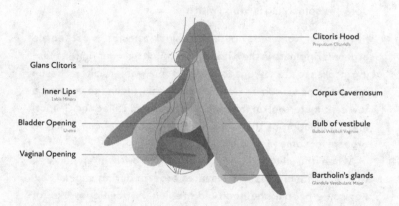

Glans Clitoris

Inner Lips
Labia Minora

Bladder Opening
Urethra

Vaginal Opening

Clitoris Hood
Preputium Clitoridis

Corpus Cavernosum

Bulb of vestibule
Bulbus Vestibuli Vaginae

Bartholin's glands
Glandula Vestibularis Major

The Clitoris: Unlike the vagina, which serves many purposes in menstruation, childbirth, and sex, the clitoris exists solely for sexual pleasure. The clitoris is the part of the body most responsible for a woman's orgasm. The nub that can be seen at the top of the vulva is only the tip of the clitoral tissue. That nub is extremely sensitive, containing more than 10,000 nerve endings. In contrast, the head of a penis has 4,000 nerve endings. So the clitoris is way more sensitive than a penis, and a touch that's too strong or direct can cause it pain. The line between pain and pleasure is delicate, which is why it is protected by its hood. The whole clitoral body is shaped like a bulbous wishbone that starts at the nub and then goes through the pelvis on the inside, along both sides of the labia. The area where clitoral tissue lies close to the top vaginal wall may create a G-spot, a sensitive area on the vaginal roof that feels very good when stimulated. The clitoral body is made of erectile tissue like a penis is, and it swells and hardens during arousal.

Rumor: You are supposed to have an orgasm from vaginal sex. I don't, so something is wrong with me.

Fact: Most women do not have vaginal orgasms. Most female orgasms originate in the clitoris from touch by a wet finger, pulsing strokes to it, a toy, or a tongue. In some women, clitoral tissue inside the pelvis comes very close to the surface of the vagina, a few centimeters in, on the roof. This has been called the G-spot, and stimulation of that area during vaginal sex can result in orgasm for some women.

When the clitoris is stimulated *along with* intercourse, a woman can more easily achieve an orgasm during vaginal sex. For some people, the good old missionary position works for this, as the pressure of the partner's pelvis rubbing against the top of the woman's vulva can stimulate the clitoris. With positions from behind, such as doggy style, the clitoris will not be stimulated unless a finger or toy is used to do so while the penis-in-vagina sex is going on.

No Shame!

If you fake pleasure during sex, don't feel bad about it. It happens! You are just doing what anyone would do if they were excited and confused, feeling pressure to "do it right" and not being sure what that even means. Your sex life is a growing and evolving thing, so don't judge yourself. Knowledge is power, so the more you learn about your body, the better sex will become for you.

Ladies First

One strategy to make sure sex is good for both the guy and the girl is to focus on the female partner's pleasure first. After she has had an orgasm stimulated by touch, oral sex, or toys, then move on to penis-in-vagina sex. Orgasm makes the clitoral tissue even more full and firm, which may then make it easier for the G-spot to be found and a vaginal orgasm to be achieved. While for most men one orgasm drains their sexual energy, women can have multiple orgasms in a single sex session. Many women feel more energized after each one.

Make Sex Less Goal Oriented

Fooling around without the goal of having an orgasm takes the pressure off. It can be fun to separate sex from orgasm and just experiment with different kinds of closeness and pleasurable touch. This kind of experimentation can expand your sexual vocabulary and help you feel more relaxed because you are not trying to achieve anything.

It's a Mental Thing

Even once a woman discovers how to orgasm and becomes familiar with her clitoris, orgasms can still sometimes be elusive. That is because there is a mental component as well. Many women find they need to deeply focus their attention on the spot being stimulated to come. They also need to be relaxed— truly, genuinely relaxed. If you are having sex while also feeling preoccupied or worried about something else, it can be hard to maintain that focus. Noise and other interruptions can distract you and kill the mood. So can worrying about getting pregnant. There are many moving parts that all have to come together to have *really good sex*. The quality of your partner, of course, and then your overall mood, setting, privacy, whether alcohol or other substances are onboard, and whether you feel confident in your birth control. Sometimes sex will just be okay, and that is fine too. It's not a contest—it's a way to feel both closeness to another person and pleasure.

FOREPLAY

Foreplay can be broken down into three stages:

1. The buildup: cultivating desire through thinking about each other, sending suggestive or romantic texts or notes, delaying gratification by spending time together and ending it with a kiss and a promise to see each other again. The thrill of randomly running into someone who really catches your eye.

2. Setting the stage: creating the romance vibe with a picnic, a sunset, a room lit by candles with soft music playing. Filling the senses with beauty.

3. Physical foreplay: long, drawn-out sessions of kisses, massage, and caresses. Taking time to explore each other's bodies while arousal builds.

Communication

It takes courage and practice to talk openly about what you like or don't like during sex. Part of it is that you are still discovering these things. Remember that it is fine to talk during sex.

If something doesn't feel good, tell your partner. If something feels amazing, give your partner encouragement! The sex act itself is a form of communication, with two bodies talking to each other. Actual words can enhance the experience.

Feeling Self-Conscious

There is not a certain age at which someone is suddenly ready for sex. Some women start in their teens and some in their 20s or even 30s. It is not a race, and there is nothing wrong with you if you do not feel ready to engage in sex. Also, sometimes you want to be sexually active for a while, and then you don't want to for a period of time. That is all normal. Health issues, life stress, and big changes can all affect how you feel about having sex. Some young people feel very self-conscious during sex. That might be a sign that they are not really ready . . . right now. Don't do it because you think you should because "everyone else is." Sex is a private, personal thing. *It's your body.* Listen to it.

Hookup Culture

Hookups are sexual encounters between partners who are not dating or in romantic relationships, with no expectation of commitment. There is a lot of theorizing about whether hookups are "good" or "bad" for women and the culture overall. Well, however good or bad they may be, hookups are definitely common. Between 60 percent and 80 percent of college students report having hookups. And like most things, it turns out there are pros and cons. In a study that began in 2014, female students were interviewed about their hookup experiences. The results of the study, "Benefits of Hooking Up: Self-Reports from First-Year College Women," were published in 2016 in the *International Journal of Sexual Health*.

In the students' own words, these were the benefits of hookups:

* Social connection
* Sexual exploration and intimacy
* Increased self-confidence
* Fun/enjoyment
* Being able to delay or avoid dating or a serious relationship and the time-consuming responsibilities that come with a serious relationship, allowing young women in college to focus more on their careers and education

These were the negative outcomes they may have experienced:

* Regretting a partner or how far it went with them sexually
* Sexual dissatisfaction
* Feelings of shame, loneliness, or embarrassment associated with STIs and sexual victimization

The bottom line is this: Hooking up is a very common practice but also an intensely personal decision. Hopefully reading what women have said about their experiences can help you decide whether it is something you want to engage in. And like everything with your sex life, you can try it, see how it feels for you, and then either continue or back off. The following chapter on consent and boundaries will help you navigate sexual encounters safely.

HOW TO MASTURBATE

1. Set and setting. You will need to be in a comfortable, private place. Your bedroom works very well, especially if you can lock the door and know that your privacy will be respected. To set the mood, you might consider turning off lights and closing curtains, lighting a candle, playing chill music.

2. Preliminary touch. Many women self-pleasure while lying on their backs with legs open. You can masturbate in any position you like, but this is a good one to start with because you can keep much of your body relaxed while you self-explore. Relaxation will enhance the experience. Take off your underwear and your clothes if that feels good. Start by lightly stroking various sensitive parts of your body—your breasts, your belly, your inner thighs. Explore what type of pressure feels most pleasant to you.

3. The genitals. As you feel more relaxed, move your hand toward your genitals and explore the lips, the vagina if that feels good, and make your way to your clitoris. Wet a finger either with spit or lube, then rub around the clit and the hood with your wet fingertip. Explore what feels good—slow and gentle; or pulsing, firm touches; or other kinds of strokes around the area. Everyone's sensations are different.

4. The mind. Once you find a kind of touch that feels pleasurable and arousing, you will need to continue this touch for a while. Close your eyes and let your mind fall to a sexual fantasy. Perhaps there is a celebrity you are crazy for—maybe a person you have a major crush on. Create a scenario that is exciting for you. Perhaps imagine them taking you into a beautiful room, undressing you, now touching and kissing you. Focus on the fantasy and keep rubbing so it feels good. As you get more aroused, you can intensify the touch and the speed.

5. Reaching climax. After a while, it might start feeling really, really good, and you may be getting close to orgasm. Orgasm feels like coming over a threshold of pleasure and then falling through. Sometimes orgasms make you tremble or shake or moan. The first time or few times, the pleasure can be very surprising—like, *I didn't know my body could feel something like that! Woah!* After orgasm, continuing to touch your clit may be too much, in which case it feels good to stop and rest. Relax and breathe into the sensations you feel.

6. Or not. Not everybody will orgasm the first time they try—new nerve pathways have to form, and it can take time. Do it until you don't want to anymore, and then stop and try again another time. Over time, your nerves will build the pathways and orgasms will become more likely.

7. Vaginal Pleasure. You can self-pleasure inside your vagina, either with (clean) fingers or a toy, such as a dildo. Experiment with fingering inside yourself, and find the places and areas that are more sensitive and pleasurable to touch. If you can wave your finger in a "come here" gesture so your fingertip strokes the roof of the vagina, you may be able to find and stimulate a very sensitive area known as the G-spot. This is where clitoral tissue comes very close to the membrane of the vaginal wall.

8. Vibrators. A powerful way to self-pleasure is with a vibrator, which can be bought at a sex shop or online. Vibrators do just that—they vibrate at various speeds, often with different settings and rhythms to explore. They cause strong sensations of pleasure and often bring a woman very rapidly to orgasm when placed next to or very near the clitoris. This can be a real breakthrough experience for people who have difficulty reaching orgasm by other means. Tips: Placing the vibrator directly on the clitoris might cause too much stimulation and be almost painful. Near or beside the clitoris is usually the best. You also can try using it through cloth or underwear to lighten the intensity.

9. Sharing. You can masturbate with your sex partner present to show them exactly how you like to be touched. Most partners find it very sexy and stimulating to watch a woman pleasure herself.

To learn more about cultivating your sexual pleasure and orgasm, I recommend the book *Come as You Are* by Emily Nagoski, PhD.

Rumor: Masturbation is bad for you, and I've heard you can go blind if you do it enough.

Fact: Many religions that place emphasis on controlling women and "keeping them in their proper place," meaning at home and submissive to their husbands, spread lies about masturbation. Providers of sexual and reproductive health care know medical research has proven that masturbation is healthy, acceptable, and safe. It has benefits in increasing sexual satisfaction for people and carries no risk.

Journal Prompts

* Reflect on what you learned about women's need for ample foreplay before sex. If you are sexually active, what things turn you on and make you feel ready for sex? Have you been satisfied with how sex has gone for you? Could you relate to any of the issues that Beth dealt with?
* Masturbation is a subject that makes some people uncomfortable, as if there is something "dirty" or "wrong" about it. This attitude actually makes it harder for women to learn

about themselves and their capacity to enjoy sex. If you had a negative reaction to the section about masturbation, write about the feelings that came up and reflect where they may have come from.

* What was the best, most romantic, most blissful experience you have had with a partner? Write about it!

Now that you have clear information about your body and its sexual pleasure, let's move into another important topic in sexual health: boundaries and consent.

10

The ABCs of a Healthy Sexual Self

Agency, Boundaries, and Consent

Agency, boundaries, and consent are the foundations of healthy relationships in all aspects of your life: family, roommates, coworkers and bosses, friends, and life/love partners. This chapter focuses on agency, consent, and boundaries when navigating sexual relationships and encounters. Having and holding clear boundaries means *not doing things we don't want to do just because others want us to*. It is something we get better at over time as we practice making and enforcing them. Many of us come from families or communities where healthy boundaries were not modeled, and if that is true for you, don't worry. You can learn about boundaries at any time in your life. Now is a great time to start.

Let's first look at what these words mean.

* *Agency* means the ability to take action or choose what action to take. In other words, when we have agency, we have control over our choices and what we do. In terms of sex, the opposite of agency is violation, in which things take place that you did not choose and you had no control over.

* *Boundaries* mark the edges between what is okay for us and
  not okay for us. We can get more familiar with our boundaries by feeling into our bodies and noticing sensations that
  communicate comfort or discomfort in response to things.
  It is hard to know what we want sometimes because there
  can be conflicting feelings, and we may not be used to listening to ourselves. But when it comes to sex, if something is
  not an enthusiastic yes, then it is a no. Learning to say no is
  a life skill that we get better at over time.
* *Consent* is agreement or permission—expressed through
  affirmative, voluntary words or actions that are mutually
  understandable to all parties involved—to engage in a
  specific sexual act at a specific time. Consent must be
  freely given and can be withdrawn at any time. Note: By
  law, consent cannot be given by someone who is underage,
  intoxicated or incapacitated by drugs or alcohol, or asleep
  or unconscious.

Agency

Agency is what we are going for in our sexual relationships;
having boundaries and using the principles of consent is how
we arrive there. Sex should feel good. There is the physical
pleasure aspect, which we touched on in the previous chapter
(pun intended), and there is the mental/emotional aspect. How
do you *feel* about the sex before, during, and after? This is more
than whether the sex was physically pleasurable—it is about
whether you felt respected as a human being. Were you listened
to, and were your needs and requests respected? Did you have
control over how things went and what transpired?

There is some confusion around this issue because there is a
common romantic fantasy of "losing control" and being "swept

off one's feet." It *is* fun to get caught up in the moment of a passionate encounter, but only if you have the agency to choose to do so and you felt a full "yes" to welcoming the experience.

Boundaries

Boundaries are the edges of what feels okay and not okay for each person. They change moment to moment and also as we grow and evolve. If you are sexually active or thinking about becoming so, it is important to explore your boundaries around sex.

If you are considering having sex with someone, reflect on the following: Why do I want to have sex? Do I feel pressured? Am I more anxious than excited? What aspects of sexual intimacy feel good to me, and what aspects make me feel awkward or uncomfortable?

Remember: You don't owe *anybody* sex. It doesn't matter if you are in a romantic relationship with someone or are already comfortable with kissing or touching them. It doesn't matter if you have previously had sex. It's also important to know that saying "I love you," buying you meals, or giving you gifts does not mean you have to have sex or do anything in return.

To develop healthy boundaries, start listening to your inner yeses and nos. For some of us, doing this is really hard! As I have mentioned elsewhere in this book, many women are raised to prioritize pleasing others over listening to and tending to their own needs. And this makes us vulnerable to victimization in sexual encounters. So, here is how to find your *no*.

Feel It in Your Gut. Your gut holds your body's wisdom. When something is a *no*, if you put your attention on your tummy, you will notice you can feel it there. That clenching sensation, that feeling of a stone sinking in there? Those are gut feelings, ways your body is signaling *no*. We can learn how to listen to ourselves, taking time to sense our feelings and developing confidence in them. If you are not sure about something, take a pause and reflect on how your body is responding to whatever is being presented to you. This is learning to notice and respect your needs and feelings. And if you aren't sure if you want to do something sexual, that is a *no*.

Sense Your No and Use It. Every day there are opportunities to feel your *yes* and *no*. For example, let's say a coworker pulls you aside at work to ask if you want to meet him for a drink over the weekend. This is a person you are not interested in getting to know outside work. How does it feel in your gut? What would you say to him? Another example: Your neighbor asks to borrow $40. But she still owes you the $60 she borrowed three months ago and never paid back. How does your gut feel when she asks for another loan? Watch for sensations of comfort and discomfort, then choose what feels right to do. What would you say to her? Remember that when people ask things of you, they are *asking*. You don't *have* to say yes. Trusting our feelings and saying no to things is how we make healthy boundaries.

Practice Asking for Consent. Try asking and not assuming. "May I take your picture?" "Would you like to share a hug?" "Can I give you a kiss?" Showing your friends and family how to ask and not assume helps to build the culture of consent. Always ask before touching someone.

Make Agreements. Practice using clear communication with a sex partner to discuss what you are comfortable with. Check in with yourself and make agreements with them before the night heats up. Do you want to just hang out and watch a show tonight? Not feeling like having sex but still want to spend time together? Interested in having sex, but only if he uses a condom? If you don't communicate what you want, then your partner will not know. Without discussion, people make assumptions about what is okay and not okay. This can lead to harm in the form of crossed boundaries.

Consent

In the world of sexual health, if it is not a *FUCK YES!!!* then it is a *no*. Meaning: When it comes to sex, if you are not over-the-moon *yes* about something, it is the safe, healthy choice to *not* do it. Sex is intimate, vulnerable, personal. It is literally baring all to someone. You are worthy of respect, of having limits, of waiting if you are not ready for something and finding alternative ways to be close. Only a *yes* means yes; everything else is a *no*. Consent is an enthusiastic YES, spoken in the absence of coercion, intimidation, or drugs or alcohol. Ambivalence, giving in to pressure, not being sure, and not being asked are all examples of not consenting. Silence is not consent. Consent is not implied by what someone is wearing or by things they have done in the past. Consent is specific to the current moment.

Hookups can carry risk because you have not built a relationship of trust with the sexual partner, so you don't know how much they will respect your boundaries, listen to you, and ask for consent. Be aware and think through what you want out of the encounter. If you can make agreements beforehand, such as that a male partner will use condoms and you will each ask permission before moving to another type of sexual touch or act, then you will have agency throughout the experience.

The Problem with Power

Unequal power dynamics—teacher and student, boss and worker, adult and underage minor—compromise our abilities to give consent. It is difficult to say no to someone who holds power over us, as we may fear the consequences of saying no. But remember, if a *no* is not available due to coercion or intimidation, it is not true consent and you are in danger of violation. If you feel your boundaries being threatened by a person in a position of power, you need to enlist support. This can be the human resources department in a workplace, the administrators at a school, or a trusted family member. You can call a rape crisis center for information about sexual harassment and what steps should be taken. Don't ignore it or face such dynamics alone.

The Problem with Age Differential and Grooming

Some older adults develop close friendships, give special gifts to, and talk about sex or share porn with underage and younger people. These behaviors are called grooming, and they are steps that may lead to that older person initiating a sexual relationship with a younger person. It is vital to watch out for grooming behaviors in the older adults in your life. You *never ever* have to allow anyone to touch you simply because they are a relative or family friend. And if you sense you are being groomed by someone, tell a trusted adult friend immediately and seek help by contacting the Rape, Abuse, and Incest National Network (RAINN) at 1-800-656-HOPE.

The Problem with Alcohol and Drugs

Someone cannot legally give consent while intoxicated by alcohol or drugs. Alcohol and recreational drugs impair people's ability to think clearly, understand facts and their implications, and make decisions. Under the influence of alcohol, people make choices they might not make if they were sober. If you are imbibing heavily, it is safer to make it a friends night and avoid pursuing sexual encounters. We are most vulnerable to harm if we are slurring words, stumbling, falling down, or sleepy. In those scenarios, it is best to get home and out of danger as swiftly as possible. Have a buddy system in which you and your friends monitor each other, and have a transportation plan, like using a ride-hailing app or a taxi, to get each other safely home.

If you are out at a bar or party and suddenly feel disoriented or much more intoxicated than you should, it is possible you have been roofied. Rohypnol, a strong sedative-hypnotic, is known as the date-rape drug. When mixed with alcohol, it causes anterograde amnesia, which means that you won't remember what happened while on the drug. Men drop it into women's drinks at bars and parties with the intention of sexually assaulting them when they are sleepy or unconscious. To prevent this, never leave your drink unattended at a bar or party. Never accept a drink or open beer from anyone. Hold on to your own drink at all times. And have an agreement with your friends that if any one of you is slurring or stumbling, they are to be taken home immediately. If one of you is very sleepy or unconscious, an ER visit is appropriate. Because of these real and all-too-common dangers, it is best not to go out to parties or a bar alone.

The Problem with Sharing Nude or Sexually Explicit Photos

It is common nowadays for men to ask, request, beg, and pressure teen girls and young women to share nude or sexually explicit/suggestive photos as part of their romantic interactions. This practice has been normalized in our age of smartphones and Snapchat. It might seem fun and flirty, and you may be flattered by their desire for your body, but *hold on a sec*. There are major issues around consent to be considered before sending someone nude photos of yourself. Too many women have become victims of cyberbullying, sextortion, and revenge porn. Before you hit Send, please understand the full ramifications of sharing nude photos of yourself with someone.

Once you have sent someone a nude photo of yourself, you have *absolutely no control* over what happens to the image afterward. It is no longer yours. It is in someone else's phone or cloud forever, regardless of the status of your relationship with them. While in theory it is illegal to post nude photos without someone's consent, in reality it happens all the time, and there is virtually no way for police or lawyers to find and penalize the person who first posted them.

Once these photos are posted on porn sites, hundreds or thousands of people might take screenshots or download the nude images, then continue to share the photos around the web. Young women find themselves the nonconsensual stars of porn sites, and like Pandora's box, they cannot scrub these pictures off the web because they just pop up elsewhere. It is a catastrophic violation that has driven some young women to suicide.

Even if you think, "I like this guy. He is so sweet, and I don't think he would ever do that to me," realize that you don't know how he might act if he gets angry or after you break up with him. People falling in love are always on their best behavior. Sometimes the person who seemed like the biggest sweetheart at first becomes an angry, aggressive ex.

If you do choose to send nude or explicit photos, have a conversation with the person you are sending them to about your boundaries and consent regarding those pictures *before* you share them. Check in with yourself after that conversation to listen for your inner *yes* or *no*.

Bringing Men into Consent Culture

If only women learn about consent, then the conversations will be pretty one-sided. Feel free to share this chapter with boyfriends, friends, brothers, and relatives. Here are some things for men as well as women to consider:

* Think of consent as obtaining a mutual agreement in which all parties are informed and free to make a voluntary choice. When we build skills of practicing consent, we shift the culture to one that affirms and respects each other's agency and autonomy.

* Men and male-identified people: Sometimes your size and your gender, as well as your age and other factors, create a power dynamic that can be intimidating for women to interact with. This can make communicating boundaries harder for them. Watch for nonverbal cues that she is experiencing discomfort and does not consent. Observe her and watch for the following: her body is leaning away from you, she is crossing her arms, or she is looking around and avoiding eye contact. Laughter can often indicate nervousness and discomfort. And of course, if she doesn't answer, it is a *no*. Silence is always a *no* and never a *yes*. Watch for these signs and, if they occur, give her space to exit the interaction with you. Step back and let her walk away. Do not pursue her if you see these nonverbal cues.

* What if someone says no to you? No can be a hard thing to hear. Turns out it is also a hard thing to say. Try not to take it personally. When someone says no, they are saying yes to themselves. They are sharing their boundaries with you,

which is a brave thing. When you get a *no*, you can try saying, "I hear you. Thank you for taking care of yourself."

* Always disclose important information, such as "I'm sick,"
  "I'm really high," "I'm being treated for an STI," or "I'm married and in an open relationship." It is not consent if you
  hide information from her.

* Remember, if she is intoxicated, she cannot freely consent,
  so give her space to leave the interaction and wait until
  another time.

* This material on consent is relevant to same-sex couples,
  nonbinary people, and transgender people. Anyone with a
  body needs to practice consent and be mindful of others'
  boundaries.

I wish I could end this chapter right here. When the patriarchy is smashed and the culture has evolved away from violence
and violation, people will be safe from sexual assault. But as
things are, if I ended the chapter here, I would be doing you a
disservice. Because sexual assault happens. One out of every
six American women have been the victim of an attempted or
completed rape. If it happens to you, you are not alone and it
is not your fault. It is the fault of patriarchy, rape culture, and
above all, the person who did it. Period.

Trigger Warning: sexual assault, sexual violence, rape, abuse,
domestic violence

Sexual Assault

"I write because the most healing words I have been
given are 'It's okay not to be okay.' It's okay to fall
apart because that's what happens when you are
broken, but I want victims to know they will not be left
there, that we will be alongside them as we rebuild."
—Chanel Miller, *Know My Name*

A Story: Recent college grad Kelsie did not realize she had been raped at age 18 until she read Chanel Miller's book, *Know My Name*. The incident happened the morning after Kelsie's 18th birthday in a hotel room with a bunch of friends. The friends had seen a concert in a big city a few hours from home and shared a hotel room afterward. She woke up to find one of her "friends" having sex with her. It was already done before she could pull her thoughts together and react.

Kelsie was sad, angry, and confused by what happened, but it was her birthday and she was with her gang. So she tried to just focus on the fun and move on. But every year on her birthday she would cry a lot and feel hopeless and traumatized. After her college graduation she read *Know My Name,* and she realized there was a name for what happened to her. It was *rape*. She began therapy to process the trauma of that experience. After about a year of therapy, as well as sharing about the experience with trusted friends and family, she felt better. Her birthday came, and she could at last celebrate it again as a joyful day.

What Is Sexual Assault and What Is Rape?

Sexual assault is any sexual contact or behavior that occurs without specific consent of the victim. It can include unwanted fondling or touch, attempted rape, rape, or forcing a victim to perform sex acts.

Rape is a form of sexual assault in which penetration of the vagina or anus occurs.

Some examples of different kinds sexual assault are:

* You are making out with someone who keeps trying to shove their fingers down your pants even though you have told them no several times.
* An established partner inserts his penis or fingers inside you while you are sleeping if you haven't given prior consent for that.
* You are in the middle of sexual intimacy with someone whom you consented to sleeping with earlier, but now something has changed. It is hurting you, or you get your period, or you change your mind. You tell them you want to stop. But they *don't*, so you try to relax and just let them get on with it.
* You get so intoxicated that you black out and wake up in bed next to someone. You don't know what happened or if you had sex, but you have bruises on your thighs.

If you have been sexually assaulted, it is likely that you carry trauma from that experience whether you realize it or not. Rape crisis counseling, therapy, and survivor support groups are important ways of beginning to heal the trauma. There is no special timeline to get help; it will benefit you whenever you start. RAINN has a 24/7 support line at 1-800-656-HOPE.

If You Are the Victim of a Rape, Here Is What to Do

Don't Blame Yourself: It is not your fault. You did not make this happen; it was beyond what you could control. It is normal to experience a range of difficult emotions, but please don't focus on blaming yourself. There was nothing you did, said, or wore that made it happen.

Get to a Safe Place: Make sure you are in a safe place or call a friend you trust to help you. Are you in immediate danger? If so, call 911. Once in a safe space, do what comforts you. You are likely in a state of both physical and emotional shock. Get in bed with warm blankets, put on soft music, have a trusted friend or family member stay by your side. Do things that are soothing to you. This will calm your nervous system and help you recover from the shock.

Consider Going to the Hospital as Soon as You Can for Two Reasons: (1) to have any injuries examined and treated, and (2) for a sexual assault forensic exam, otherwise known as a rape kit.

A Note on Rape Kits: Many victims of rape are reluctant to go to a hospital after an assault, and the decision is up to you. You may not know if you want to press charges or talk to the police at the moment, but you can still have the evidence collected. For the most accurate rape kit, it is best if you don't wash the area, shower, change clothes, or do anything to alter yourself first. If you are not ready to face the hospital, you can wait. The assault exam can be done up to 72 hours after the incident, even if you wash and change. But if you do that, there will be less DNA found. In this case, you can bring the clothes you were wearing to the hospital in a bag.

Medical Care: If you are not currently on a form of birth control, get an emergency contraceptive pill from the hospital, a clinic, or over the counter from a drugstore and take it as soon as possible, within 72 hours of the assault.

If you choose not to get immediate medical care, follow up as soon as you can at a reproductive health clinic or gynecologist/midwife office. The clinic, provider, or midwife will provide STI testing, and then you can repeat the testing in four weeks. They will also offer you prophylactic treatment for chlamydia and/or gonorrhea. Prophylactic means they will treat you right away, just based on your history of possibly being exposed, without waiting for test results.

If you are concerned about exposure to HIV, you can discuss a medication regimen called post-exposure prophylaxis (PEP) with your doctor or provider. It must be started within 72 hours of exposure and is taken daily for a month. Research suggests that PEP can reduce your chances of contracting HIV by up to 80 percent.

Seek Support: You will need help healing from the trauma of the assault. Call a rape crisis center for initial support. RAINN has a 24/7 support line at 1-800-656-HOPE. Many communities have their own rape crisis centers and hotlines.

Survivors of sexual assault might experience depression, anxiety, dissociation, and other mental health issues over time. Consider therapy or other ongoing survivor services. Remember, it is normal to need extra support when recovering from a sexual assault. And it is very hard to process such a difficult experience without professional help from a counselor or therapist. As Miller wrote in *Know My Name*, "It's okay not to be okay."

Heal the trauma on your own timeline. There is no standard schedule for healing the trauma from sexual assault and rape. Every person does it at their own pace. For some people, it takes years before they are ready to acknowledge the assault, while others may want to start processing the trauma right away. There is no wrong way to heal. So be gentle on yourself and don't feel rushed or pressured to do anything about it. You will know when you are ready.

Final Considerations: Partner Abuse and Domestic Violence

Not all abuse from partners is sexual. Some partners might be physically or emotionally abusive. People who abuse do so out of an extreme need to control others. Any person who has abused you will abuse you again, even if they are very sorry about it afterward. And even if it only happens sometimes or rarely. No matter how much you may love them, they will not be safe for you to stay in a relationship with. Next I'm going to share some examples of abusive behavior.

Physical Abuse: Anything that involves physical force, such as hitting, breaking things, throwing things, pushing, shoving, committing sexual assault, damaging material possessions, or using their bodies to block or physically intimidate.

Emotional Abuse: Behavior that inflicts psychological harm or mental distress. Examples include threats of violence or harm, yelling and shouting, calling someone names, using degrading or demeaning language with them, using manipulation tactics to control them, or gaslighting them. Gaslighting is a type of behavior in which a partner undermines someone and makes them lose confidence in themselves in order to control them. An example of gaslighting is if a partner insists that you are being irrational when you bring up something you're upset about instead of addressing that issue.

If you are concerned about your own safety or the safety of someone else involved in a dangerous relationship, call the National Domestic Violence Hotline: 1-800-799-7233.

Journal Prompts and Reflections

* Are there things you struggle with saying no to? What are the fears that might be keeping you from saying no? What do you think would happen if you said no?
* Describe a time you felt respected. What did communication look like before, during, and after that interaction?
* Now describe a time you felt disrespected. What did communication look like before, during, and after that interaction?
* Describe a time you had a gut feeling about something or someone. What took place and how did you handle that? After learning about boundaries, what would you do the next time you had a similar feeling?

* Has anyone asked for nude photos of you? How did you feel about that? How might you handle it in the future after reading about the risks of sharing explicit photos?

Further Resources

If you or someone you know is a victim of sexual harassment or sexual assault:
* National Sexual Assault Hotline (1-800-656-4673; www.rainn.org)
* National Sexual Violence Resource Center (www.nsvrc.org/find-help)
* Chanel Miller, *Know My Name* (New York: Viking, 2019)

If you are a victim of cybercrime or revenge porn:
* Cyber Civil Rights Initiative Crisis Helpline (1-844-878-2274; cybercivilrights.org/ccri-crisis-helpline)
* www.helpguide.org/dealing-with-revenge-porn-and-sextortion
* fightcybercrime.org/scams/harassment/revenge-porn/

If you are under 18 and someone has posted nude photos of you on the internet:
* National Center for Missing & Exploited Children (takeitdown.ncmec.org)
* Childhelp National Child Abuse Hotline (1-800-4-A-CHILD; 1-800-422-4453)

11

The Empowered Approach to Unintended Pregnancy

High school student Claire had sex with her first boyfriend a few times. She was going to get on birth control, but she wasn't that worried about it. She thought maybe she couldn't get pregnant, as her periods were not regular. She missed one period, which was not that unusual for her. Then she missed another one and realized she hadn't had a period in almost three months. One morning, the smell of scrambled eggs made her run to the bathroom, gagging. That night she took three at-home pregnancy tests from the dollar store, and they all came back positive.

College sophomore Nadine was on the pill and had been for a couple of years. She went on a spring break trip with her partner and forgot to bring her pills. She figured she had been on pills for so long she was probably still safe. She got back and waited for her period to come, to start a new pack, but it never came. Her boyfriend bought a pregnancy test and brought it to her. They were both shocked to see it turn positive.

Twenty-four-year-old Jolie (almost) always used condoms.

She didn't like birth control; she had tried several kinds over the years. She knew exactly the night it happened. She hooked up with a guy she used to date, and for some reason, they didn't use a condom. She was moving out of her apartment that weekend, and in the chaos of packing, she forgot to take a Plan B as well. She thought the missed period was caused by the stress of moving, but when she noticed that her breasts were very tender, she took a pregnancy test. It was positive.

Unintended pregnancy happens. According to the latest statistics, three out of 10 women will get pregnant before age 20, and 80 percent of those pregnancies will be unintended. In my clinic, I have seen women get pregnant while on the pill, even while using it correctly. I have seen women get pregnant with an IUD in place. And I have seen women who gave birth recently, shocked to be pregnant again within two months of the delivery. If it happens to you, know that you are not alone. You will need to decide what to do, but that does not need to happen immediately. The following four steps are an empowered approach to unintended pregnancy:

1. Confirm the pregnancy. Otherwise, you may think you are pregnant and not be!
2. Feel the feels. It is important to give space for the emotions that come up after finding out you're pregnant. You might feel shock, disbelief, worry, excitement, anger, or ambivalence. Feelings can change rapidly, day to day and hour to hour, as your mind processes the information that you are pregnant. These feelings are normal; let them be. Just don't get stuck in self-blame. If you have a friend or family member you trust to be confidential and nonjudgmental, it can help to talk to someone.
3. Learn about your options. Knowledge is power, and you

need to know what your choices are before you make one.
An *option* is a thing that is or may be chosen. The following
chapters provide information on each option.

4. Decide what is right for *you*. Your partner, boyfriend,
spouse, family, or friends should not decide what to do.
They should not pressure you or tell you what to do. You are
the only person who is pregnant in this situation, and you
are the only person who should choose what to do. If people
are pressuring you, you may have to take space from them
to filter out the noise and listen to what feels right to *you*.
Spend time alone in your room, sit by a creek or body of
water, or take a long walk in nature before you decide. If you
listen to other people and not yourself, you are more likely
to experience regret.

Confirm the Pregnancy

If you think you might be pregnant, the first thing to do is take a
pregnancy test. Urine pregnancy tests are simple, accurate tests
that detect a pregnancy hormone called human chorionic gonado-
tropin (HCG) if it is circulating in your body. HCG can be detected
in your urine before you have any other signs of pregnancy.

Pregnancy tests can be purchased at any drugstore, and even
dollar stores carry them. Each pregnancy test is slightly different, so you will need to follow the package instructions. For all
of them, you will:

1. Pee into a cup.
2. Dip a test strip in the urine for a specific number of seconds,
per the package instructions.
3. Set the strip down on a flat surface and wait—usually three
to five minutes—to read the results. Every test strip has

room for two lines: the C line, which stands for *control* and will always be present unless the test is invalid, and the T line, which stands for *test*. This line only turns up if there is HCG in your urine. If, after the allotted time, the T line is absent, the test result is negative. You can take another test in a few days if your period still has not come. If there is a T line, the test is positive.

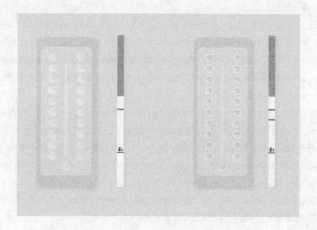

I think I might have gotten pregnant this month. When should I take a pregnancy test?

A pregnancy test will not come back positive until two weeks after conception, which for most women is about a day after your period should have started. The timing of getting pregnant looks something like this:

Your last period started on day 1 of a 28-day "month."

Ovulation occurs at approximately day 14 (two weeks *after* the first day of your last period). Conception can occur within a few days on either side of ovulation. This is because sperm can live inside you for a few days, and the viable egg is present for about 48 hours after ovulation.

Between day 14 and day 28, a fertilized egg will float through your fallopian tube and into the uterus, where it will implant into the uterine lining and start developing. While it is floating, it does not make HCG that can be detected in your bloodstream or by a pregnancy test.

Implantation occurs around day 28 (four weeks after the first day of your last period). Your period is expected but does not come because the fertilized egg arrives in the uterus and embeds itself into the uterine lining. This signals the lining to stay put and not slough off. The embryo, placenta, and gestational sac begin to form. At this point the levels of HCG in your blood and urine start doubling every 48 hours and will continue to do so until you are about 10 weeks along. You will get a positive pregnancy test if you take one.

Remember, a pregnancy test will not be positive until implantation has occurred. So you cannot take one the day after you think you may have gotten pregnant. (You *can* take a morning-after pill, however.) Missing your period is usually the first sign of a pregnancy and is also when you can get an accurate pregnancy test result. Tracking your cycles with an app can help you stay aware of when your period should arrive.

Early Signs of Pregnancy

Missed Period: Occurs four weeks after last period. Sometimes there can be light spotting when implantation happens, with no other menstrual symptoms. But it is not heavy and does not last for several days like your normal period.

Fatigue: Occurs five to six weeks after the last period. Some women experience deep, bone-level fatigue during early pregnancy. Some may sleep 10 to 12 hours a night when seven to eight hours is their nonpregnant norm.

Breast Tenderness and Other Breast Changes: Starts four to six weeks after the last period. Unusual breast tenderness is a common first sign of pregnancy, along with a missed period. The breasts can become so sensitive that a friend's hug can send shocking sensations of pain through you. Your breasts might grow a cup size or more in the first months of pregnancy.

Nausea and Vomiting: Starts five to seven weeks after the last period. This pregnancy symptom is commonly called "morning sickness," although it can occur any time of day. Triggers can be an empty stomach, low blood sugar, or certain smells, especially the smell of food cooking. Keeping crackers at the bedside to eat as soon as you wake up or nibbling protein snacks throughout the day can help relieve nausea.

Note: Everyone's body is different. Some women have none of these symptoms except the missed period, and some have all of them. And each pregnancy is different, even for the same woman.

I got a positive pregnancy test at home. I'm not sure what I want to do. Now what?

If there is any chance that you are going to continue the pregnancy, remember that anything you put in your body is also going to get to the developing fetus. Please consider the following:

* Stop drinking alcohol. Alcohol is highly toxic to a developing fetus, and its use during pregnancy can cause irreversible mental impairments and birth defects.

* Quit smoking, which can cause low birthweight, premature delivery, and other pregnancy complications. Call 1-800-QUIT-NOW for help.

* Stop taking birth control pills if you are on them. If you use the patch or ring, take them off/out.

* Avoid medicines and drugs, and check with a health care provider about prescription medications you take.

* Be sure to let any doctor or dentist that you see for other reasons know that you are pregnant. It may be safer to delay or change plans for medical and dental procedures or treatments.

* Take folic acid, eat fresh fruits and vegetables, and get plenty of sleep.

I have been partying a lot lately and didn't know I was pregnant. Did I mess up my chance to have a healthy pregnancy?

Nope, as long as you stop partying now. During the first two weeks after conception, when the fertilized egg is on the move through the fallopian tube, the pregnancy is not exposed to what you take, eat, or drink. It is not until implantation that exposure begins. The sooner you stop, the better. If you are having a hard time stopping drug or alcohol use and you want to continue the pregnancy, you may need professional substance abuse recovery services.

The next step is to go to a clinic, health department, or doctor's office and take a pregnancy test there to confirm the pregnancy, get counseling about your options, and obtain resources and referrals for further services.

If you have already been seen at a clinic for birth control or STI testing in the past, that is a good place to go for the pregnancy confirmation. You can also go to an OB/GYN's office, although they may be biased and not counsel you on the full range of pregnancy options, especially in states where abortions are legally limited. Planned Parenthood has clinics throughout the country and is always a good bet. You can go to a Planned Parenthood or other reproductive health clinic to confirm your pregnancy regardless of what you decide to do about it.

Beware of Fake Clinics: Crisis pregnancy centers are offices that look like and advertise themselves as real reproductive health clinics, but they're not. They are run by antiabortion activists and may not have any real medical professionals on staff. They are dishonest and use deception, shaming tactics, manipulation, and pressure to dissuade women from accessing abortion services or even from using birth control. They often set up near real clinics, such as a Planned Parenthood, and dress up like health professionals—in white lab coats and scrubs, for example—to trick pregnant people. They don't follow medical confidentiality laws either, and they might give your personal information to antiabortion organizations to further harass you.

These fake clinics often call themselves pregnancy help centers, pregnancy resource centers, or pregnancy care centers. They offer free pregnancy testing and abortion "counseling" but don't actually offer abortions. They may even have ultrasounds in-house to date your pregnancy, but they might use the technology to confuse you about when you could safely have an abortion. They rob you of your rights to information and your access to health services. They are also dangerous because they are likely to miss complications or abnormalities, such as ectopic pregnancy, that a legitimate health care provider would catch. There are 3,000 fake clinics in the United States. To check in your area and ensure you are going to a legitimate reproductive health clinic, visit the following websites:

exposefakeclinics.com
crisispregnancycentermap.com
The Fake Clinic Database at reproaction.org/fakeclinicdatabase

At a legitimate reproductive health clinic, doctor/midwife office, or health department, you will take another urine pregnancy test, just like you did at home. However, a nurse or other health professional will read the result, then help you determine how far along you are based on the date of your last period. If you don't know when your last period was, the clinic may offer you a physical exam or an ultrasound.

A human pregnancy lasts approximately 40 weeks from the first day of a last period. You will be given an estimated due date and told how many weeks pregnant you are. But remember, the first two weeks of that you weren't pregnant yet, and the following two weeks was the phase between conception and implantation. So if you are told you are six weeks along, it has only been two weeks since implantation. A bit confusing, isn't it? With an estimated due date established, the clinic can give you the paperwork you need to obtain referrals, pregnancy-only Medicaid insurance if you are uninsured, and other resources. They also should counsel you about your options.

I Am Pregnant.
What Are My Options?

You have three options. They are:

1. Continue the pregnancy, have and raise the baby
2. Continue the pregnancy and place the baby for adoption
3. End the pregnancy by having an abortion

You don't have to decide right away. But if you might continue the pregnancy, it is best to follow the health recommendations listed on pages 167 and 168. Also, you need to be aware that there are time limits to accessing abortion, especially medical abortion, which is best done under 10 weeks gestation by last menstrual period. It is *very important* you sit with the decision until you feel clear about what you want to do. And it is very important that no one pressures you or tries to make you do something. *It's your pregnancy.* The following chapters provide both medical and logistic facts about each option, as well as stories shared by women who have made these choices before you. That way, you can get a sampling of women's real-life experiences with all the options.

Special Consideration: Miscarriage

One out of four early pregnancies spontaneously ends in a miscarriage, usually within the first couple of months. If you miscarry, it is not your fault and it is not the result of anything you have done. It is likely that the pregnancy was not developing normally, and early miscarriage is Mother Nature's way of cleaning house. If you have a positive pregnancy test and then begin cramping, with bleeding as heavy as or heavier than a period, you may be miscarrying. It is safe to stay home and pass an early pregnancy by yourself. But you need to be seen in an ER if you:

* Bleed too heavily, which is defined by filling a large maxi pad every 30 minutes for more than two hours
* Develop a fever
* Feel faint or pass out
* Have severe pain

Most women who miscarry in early pregnancy do not have complications, but there can be grief and a sense of loss afterward. To help with post-miscarriage grief or depression, I recommend following up with a midwife or at a clinic and joining a support group for pregnancy loss. After a miscarriage, a pregnancy test will still be positive for about four weeks, as the pregnancy hormones are still in your system. After four weeks have passed, a pregnancy test should be negative.

Journal Prompts/Reflections

When thinking about parenting, adoption, and abortion, consider the following questions:

* How would my decision affect my future, my family, my other children?
* Am I ready to go through pregnancy and childbirth?
* Am I ready to raise a child?
* Do I have strong personal or religious beliefs about parenting, adoption, or abortion?
* Would anyone pressure me to make a certain choice?
* Will my family, friends, or partner support me?
* Who can I talk to about facing this decision? Who would be understanding and not judge me?

12

Your Pregnancy, Your Options

Option #1

Continuing the Pregnancy, Having the Baby, Raising the Child

Am I Ready to Raise a Child?

This is a question only you can answer. Raising a child is both one of the most fulfilling things a person will ever do and a monumental undertaking that will impact every facet of your life. Family, relationships, money, life goals, personal beliefs, and the well-being of the future child are all things people consider when choosing to become a parent. The good news is that you don't have to figure everything out *now*. Child-rearing is a long-term project, and even people who planned their pregnancy will figure things out as they go. No one is ever completely ready to have a child, but that shouldn't keep you from doing it if you want to. To get a future child off to a good start now, what you need is:

* A safe environment for you to live in, free from physical and emotional harm

* The ability to take care of your own health and well-being,
  which then takes care of the growing pregnancy. The basics
  of taking care of yourself: doing your best not to smoke,
  drink, or use other substances; taking a prenatal vitamin;
  eating a diet rich in fresh foods, especially proteins, fruits,
  and vegetables; and getting adequate rest
* Prenatal care
* A support network of family and/or friends to help you after
  the baby arrives while you are recovering from the birth
  and learning how to take care of your new baby
* A plan for financial support after the birth for yourself and
  your child. Will someone support you or will you work?
  Will you go to school? If you work or attend school, who
  will care for the baby while you are there?

Everything will come, one step at a time.

Prenatal Care

It is important to establish care with a prenatal health care provider. Prenatal care consists of specialized health checkups to make
sure you and the developing fetus are healthy. With the paperwork
from the clinic or health department that verifies your pregnancy,
you can apply for Medicaid pregnancy-only health insurance and
get an appointment for prenatal care. You can also get into a nutrition program called WIC (women, infants, and children) for free or
low-cost foods. Your prenatal provider can refer you to education
programs, such as childbirth and parenting classes.

You can choose whether a doctor or a midwife cares for you
during your pregnancy, even if you have Medicaid. So it is important you know the difference between a doctor and a midwife.

OB/GYNs are surgeons and experts in disease management. They provide prenatal care to healthy pregnant women, but the visits are usually brief and focus on lab test results, physical exams, and measurements. They are excellent at managing high-risk pregnancies, such as pregnant women with diabetes, high blood pressure, twins, heart disease, or preterm labor.

Eighty percent of pregnant women are healthy and are good candidates for midwifery care. The word *midwife* means "with woman," and midwives take a more holistic approach to prenatal care. This means they support the whole woman through the changes of pregnancy, birth, and the transition to parenthood. Midwives offer the same medical testing as doctors, but appointments are usually longer and include time to talk and address the emotional, psychological, and social changes of the pregnancy. They help you plan for your birth and the postpartum period and are experts in natural childbirth. In many places around the country, women with Medicaid insurance and private insurance can see hospital-based nurse-midwives for their care during pregnancy and birth, with doctors available in case health complications develop. There are also home birth midwives for women who prefer to give birth in their own homes. Home birth midwives may or may not take insurance but usually have payment plans or financial assistance programs.

Many women find their prenatal providers through word of mouth in their communities. You can do an internet search for OB/GYNs and midwives in your area, then set up interviews to meet them before selecting one. That way, you can select a provider you trust and like.

Questions to ask a potential prenatal care provider (either doctor or midwife) include:

* How long have you been in practice, and how many babies have you delivered?

* Will I be seeing you for all my prenatal appointments?

* Who will deliver the baby? Are you part of a big call group, or do you come for your own deliveries?

* What is your Cesarean section rate? Under what circumstances would you do one?

* How do you accommodate people's birth plan preferences?

* Would you be comfortable if I brought a doula or labor support person to the birth with me?

* What do you like about being an OB/midwife?

Did you feel respected and listened to by the midwife or doctor? Did you sense you were being judged for being young or for any other reason, or did you leave the visit feeling good about yourself? Use what you have learned about agency, respect, and boundaries in chapter 10 to choose your care provider during this important time in your life. If you didn't get a good gut feeling from the visit, it's okay to find a different provider.

Option #2

Continuing the Pregnancy, Placing the Baby for Adoption

Placing a child for adoption is a parenting choice made with the well-being of the child in mind. It is a loving, responsible choice for a birth mother who feels she cannot parent the child, whatever the reasons may be.

Some reasons a pregnant person may choose to place a baby for adoption are:

* They aren't ready or are too young to parent a child.
* They can't give a child the life they would want for them. Single motherhood, lack of stability and support, substance addiction, and domestic violence are examples of life situations that may not be congruent with raising a child.
* They have religious or spiritual reasons for choosing adoption over abortion.
* They want control over when and with whom they start a family.
* They don't have access to abortion or are too far along in the pregnancy.
* They know there is a family out there who would raise the baby the way they would want them to be raised, even if they could not. Also, they get to pick that family for the child.

Placing a Child, Not Giving Up a Child

You are neither "giving up" the baby nor "giving it away." A birth mother who decides to place her child for adoption chooses a family for the child, but she will always remain the birth mother of the child. Adoption is *not* child abandonment; it is another way of providing for the child.

What Exactly Is Involved?

Most adoptions are now planned as open adoptions. This means that the birth parents have the opportunity to participate fully in their adoption plan, including selecting the parents they believe to be best for their child; meeting, interviewing, and getting to know the adoptive parents; sharing information with the adoptive parents; spending time with the baby while in the hospital; deciding whether to have ongoing contact with the adoptive family and child; and negotiating the type of ongoing contact desired, such as letters, pictures, or visits. Adoption programs support your right to an open relationship with the adoptive family, if you choose, and will offer you guidance and support. Not all birth parents feel comfortable with open adoption, and it doesn't have to be open. The choice is always up to *you*.

If you think that placing the child for adoption may be the right option for you, the first step is to contact an adoption program or adoption service provider. Your local clinic, health department, or OB/GYN should be able to put you in contact with the adoption program for your area.

The adoption program will provide:

* Information about the process
* Counseling to ensure you fully understand your decision and your rights as a birth mother
* Facilitation of the adoption
* Support and advocacy
* Assistance with practical support, such as helping fund

your housing, transportation costs, prenatal care, and other pregnancy-related needs

Adoption services are:

* Confidential. Even if you choose open adoption, all services are private and confidential. You do not need your parents' consent to seek adoption.
* Free. Adoption services are free to birth parents. Additionally, appropriate costs related to your pregnancy can be paid for by the adoptive parents.
* Helpful. They will find supportive and appropriate medical care, even if you are late in your pregnancy.
* Protective of your legal rights. You can change your mind at any time, and the final consents are not signed until after the child's birth. In most states you will have time even after you place the baby with the adoptive parents to decide whether you have made the right decision.

How Does Picking a Family Work?

In a typical open adoption, you will be asked to look through files on all the people looking to adopt. There are many diverse families eagerly waiting to adopt a child. In their files, you will be able to see their photographs and read about them—where they live, what they do, what they like, how they would like to raise a child, whether they have other children, their religious beliefs, and their ideas about adoption. You select the people you would like to find out more about. Then, if you want to, the program will set up a time for you to meet them to see if they are the people you want to raise your child. When you decide, an adoption service provider will meet with you to advise you of your rights and responsibilities.

Shortly before your due date, the adoption program meets with you and your adoptive family to discuss how you want things to go at the hospital and what your desires are for contact with the child and adoptive family after the birth and placement. The baby can go directly home from the hospital with the adoptive family. After the birth, you will meet your adoption service provider again to sign a placement agreement, which becomes your final consent 30 days after you sign it. In some states this timeline may be different. Within 8 to 10 months, the adoptive parents will go to court to finalize the adoption.

Considerations

There is loss and grief inherent in this choice, as well as joy and excitement. It is normal to feel loss after placing a child for adoption, even if you know this was the best possible decision for that child. It is a tender moment to leave the hospital without the baby after giving birth. The adoption stories in the next chapter describe the experience and the spectrum of emotions birth mothers typically feel, including grief, peace, relief, happiness, and pride in themselves for their brave choice. Most adoption programs include counseling and social support for the birth mother throughout the process and after.

Option #3

Ending the Pregnancy by Having an Abortion

Abortion is a medical process that ends a pregnancy. Some reasons women might choose to have an abortion are:

* Not ready or prepared for motherhood
* Wants control over when and with whom they have a child
* Does not desire a child
* Already has a child/children and struggles to provide for or focus on them
* Current lifestyle not compatible with parenting
* Current life stage not conducive to motherhood (examples: in middle of education, doesn't have stable housing, far from home, or lacking family support)
* Relationship problems, abusive partner, or no partner and does not want to be a single mother
* Has been a victim of sexual assault that resulted in pregnancy

There are two types of abortion. They are:

Surgical Abortion, or Uterine Suction Aspiration: Can be done in most settings that provide abortions up to 14 weeks, and in some settings it is available to 24 weeks.

Medical Abortion, or Abortion Pills: Medical abortion care can be provided by in-person care or telemedicine, or it can be self-managed. It currently can be done up to 10 weeks in the United

States, but that may be extended soon to 12 weeks based on World Health Organization guidelines.

What Is Surgical Abortion?

First of all, surgical abortion is not actually *surgery* because nothing on or in your body is cut. It is a gynecologic *procedure*. During surgical abortion, a tube is admitted through the opening (os) in the cervix and into the uterus, and the pregnancy tissue is removed from the uterus by suction. The procedure itself takes about 10 minutes, although you will likely spend a couple of hours to half a day in pre-care and post-care at the clinic.

Surgical abortion is one of the safest medical procedures that exists. Approximately 98 percent of them have no complications. When there are complications, such as bleeding or infection, a short course of medication or a repeat of the procedure will resolve the problem. There are no long-term health problems, such as infertility or increased risk of cancer, associated with surgical abortion.

Surgical abortion can be accomplished from six weeks of pregnancy up until 24 weeks of pregnancy. However, most clinics that offer them provide them up to about 14 weeks of pregnancy. If you are further along than that, you may have to be referred to a larger or more specialized facility.

For most surgical abortions, women are given oral medications for pain, anxiety, and nausea. Some facilities offer IV medications for pain and sedation, especially at sites where later second trimester abortions are performed. You will come to the clinic a couple of hours before your procedure for counseling and medication.

During the procedure, the doctor will:

1. Insert a speculum into your vagina to view the cervix
2. Clean your cervix and vagina with gauze soaked in soap/antiseptic

3. Apply numbing medication to your cervix
4. Dilate your cervical os, the tight opening to your uterus, with a series of thin rods
5. Insert a narrow, flexible tube into your uterus
6. Apply gentle suction to the other end of the tube to remove the pregnancy tissue

Toward the end of the procedure, you may feel a cramp similar to a menstrual cramp in your uterus as it shrinks down to a nonpregnant size. The doctor can insert an IUD for you right after the suction tube is removed if you want one.

Right after the procedure, you will rest in an aftercare room. You may be given a heating pad, warm blankets, juice or something to drink, and snacks. When you feel ready to get up, you will use the restroom, check your bleeding, check in with the nurse, and then go home, usually about 45 minutes after the procedure. Bleeding is usually minimal, like a heavy period for a couple of days, and then light on-and-off spotting for up to two weeks after. Many clinics will send you home with birth control to start if you want it, and it is advised to wait two weeks to have sex, or until your bleeding has completely stopped. And be careful because you can get pregnant after an abortion before you have a period.

Is Surgical Abortion Legal Where I Live?

Up until June 2022, surgical abortion was legal in all 50 states. Since the *Dobbs* decision, which ended federal protection of the right to an abortion, it is now up to each state. Some states are now limiting and banning abortions, and the legal landscape is changing all the time. You will need to find out what is legal in your state and make a plan. Because state laws are changing rapidly, I recommend using the website abortionfinder.org to check the status of abortion in your state or region. As of the end of 2023:

States with a Near-Total Abortion Ban Are: Alabama, Arkansas, Idaho, Kentucky, Louisiana, Mississippi, Missouri, Oklahoma, South Dakota, Tennessee, Texas, Indiana, North Dakota, and West Virginia.

States with Various Limits, Some of Which Are Currently Challenged in Court Are: Florida, Utah, Arizona, Nebraska, North Carolina, South Carolina, and Georgia.

States with No Clinics for Abortion Services Are: North Dakota.

What Am I Supposed to Do if I Live in One of These States and Want to Have an Abortion?

If you live in a state where abortion is limited or banned, you can:

* Travel out of state to have a surgical abortion: Go to abortionfinder.org to find the closest locations of vetted and safe abortion providers.
* Have a medical abortion, either by traveling out of state for in-person or telehealth services, or where you are via self-managed abortion services accessed online.

If you are not sure of abortion's legal standing in your state, abortionfinder.org is the place to start. After you put in your location and how far along you are, AbortionFinder provides the current legal status of medical and surgical abortion in your state and lists all your options for accessing abortion services.

To make your online search confidential, you can use Duck-DuckGo as your search engine and use the app Signal to make your calls.

What Is Medical Abortion?

Medical abortion is a series of pills that cause the pregnancy to end and your body to expel it. The expulsion takes place over several hours of uterine cramping and vaginal bleeding, making the process similar to a miscarriage. Medical abortion usually takes place in one's own home or other private and comfortable space of your choice. Since *Roe v. Wade* was overturned in June 2022, it has become the more common type of abortion in the United States.

Medical abortion is used in the United States up until 10 to 13 weeks of pregnancy, depending on the provider. This type of abortion works 93 percent to 95 percent of the time. In 5 percent to 7 percent of women, it does not completely work, and those women will need a surgical abortion or a hospital procedure called a dilatation and curettage (D&C) to finish removing the pregnancy tissue.

The pills for a medical abortion can be obtained in person at a clinic, via telemedicine in states where abortion is legal, or through online/mail services.

Who Can Use Medical Abortion Pills?

Medical abortion pills should only be taken if you are less than 13 weeks along. They are best used by women who are sure of their last menstrual period or have had other diagnostic pregnancy dating, such as an early ultrasound. When these medicines are prescribed by telemedicine or purchased online for self-managed medical abortion, it is up to the woman herself to know how far along she is (hello, cycle-tracking apps). Taking these pills if you are beyond the 10 to 13 weeks is not necessarily dangerous, but they likely will not work.

There are a few medical conditions that make medical abortion pills an unsafe choice. They are bleeding disorders, adrenal disease or failure, porphyrias, a history of obstetric hemorrhage, long-term corticosteroid use, a known allergy to these medications, or if you have an IUD in place. If any of these conditions describe you, you need to see a doctor about your situation.

You should take the pills in a location not more than an hour from a hospital emergency room and know how to get there if needed. If you are uncertain about the legal status of abortion where you are located and you need to go to a hospital for complications, you can say: "I am having a miscarriage." There is no test to detect the medical abortion medications in your system, and the treatment is exactly the same regardless of whether the miscarriage is spontaneous or medication-induced.

Where Can I Get a Medical Abortion?

Reproductive health activists and clinicians have worked hard to make medical abortion available to people in all 50 states. If abortion services are not available through an in-person clinic where you live, I recommend going to the website, www. plancpills.org. On that website, you enter your state and will be given resources for online clinics that mail abortion pills, websites that sell pills, and community networks that mail pills. The safety, cost, and legal considerations of each service listed are addressed. Remember you can use the search engine Duck, Duck Go to keep your internet search confidential.

HOW TO TAKE MEDICAL ABORTION PILLS

It is very important that you follow the instructions and take the pills correctly. You will receive:

* One pill of mifepristone, or Mifeprex
* Four small white pills of misoprostol, or Cytotec

Some providers also provide anti-nausea pills, such as Vistaril. Nausea is a common side effect of misoprostol. Anti-nausea pills can also be helpful if you are having pregnancy-related nausea and vomiting. You can also buy Unisom or other OTC anti-nausea medications at a drugstore or pharmacy.

The two medications are taken on separate days, between 24 and 48 hours apart. The bleeding and cramping occur after you have taken the second set of medications. To prepare for the abortion, you should have a private, comfortable room with a bathroom, fluids to sip and stay hydrated throughout the process, a heating pad for comfort, and a package of large maxi pads.

Step 1. Take the single mifepristone (Mifeprex) pill. This medication stops the pregnancy from growing but does not make it come out. Women usually have minimal effects after taking this pill, although some occasionally note a small amount of spotting.

Step 2. Wait 24 to 48 hours. You can do your normal activities, work, attend school, and prepare what you need for the day you take misoprostol.

Step 3. You will use *all four pills at once*. Put two of the misoprostol pills on each side of your mouth. Place them in the pouch between your inner cheek and your lower gum (like a chipmunk). There will be two on each side—so the four pills are in your mouth at once. Keep the pills in your lower cheeks for 30 minutes—set a timer. At the end of the 30 minutes, drink water and swallow the remainder of the pills.

Bleeding and cramping will start within a half hour to three hours after swallowing the pills. It will start as light bleeding and then progress to heavy bleeding with cramping. Some women experience the cramping as intense and painful, while others find it's not as bad as they thought it would be. Each person's experience is different. You can take 600 mg of ibuprofen every four to six hours for pain and use a heating pad. Do not get in a tub bath or submerge in water, but feel free to stand in a hot shower if that helps. The bleeding will progress until you are soaking a maxi pad every half hour. After one to two hours of heavy bleeding, you should pass the pregnancy, which will look like a clump of clots, but you may see the membrane of the gestational sac or the placenta. Sometimes women see and can identify the embryo but not always. Women usually sit on the toilet when the bleeding is very heavy and pass the pregnancy there.

Once the pregnancy has passed, the bleeding and cramping will lighten. If you take the medications midday, by the time you go to bed 10 hours later, the bleeding should be like a heavy period. You will bleed for the next two weeks, and it will get lighter over that time. *To prevent infection, it is very important that you do not put anything inside your vagina.* So you must wear pads and not use tampons for the full two weeks.

COMPLICATIONS

Rare but potentially serious complications can occur with medical abortion. You need to know what the signs of these complications are and that you must seek medical attention if they occur. If left untreated they can be life-threatening to you. These signs are too much bleeding and uterine infection. Be mindful if you have:

* Prolonged heavy bleeding, in which you have fully soaked a pad every 30 minutes for four hours

* A temperature of over 100.4 degrees, feeling feverish and flu-like with chills and body aches, lower abdominal tenderness, nausea and vomiting that won't stop, or severe pain anywhere, other than uterine cramping

If the above signs occur, you must get medical help. If you obtained the pills through a provider, clinic, or telehealth service, call their emergency number for instructions. If you are doing a self-managed abortion, you can call the Miscarriage + Abortion hotline for advice at 1-833-246-2632. If you have either of the above danger signs, you may need to go to an emergency room. You may be worried about going for help if abortion is not legal where you are, *but you still must go*. If you fear legal prosecution, use the words, "I am having a miscarriage," then tell them about the bleeding or fever. As I stated above, the medications are not detectable by blood test or any kind of testing.

The good news is that the most common complication of medical abortion is not life-threatening and not an emergency that requires a hospital visit. In 5 percent to 7 percent of medical abortions, the abortion is incomplete and some pregnancy tissue remains in the body. Signs that you may not have completely passed the pregnancy are:

✶ You did not have bleeding heavier than a period and you did not pass any clots or tissue.

✶ You still have pregnancy symptoms, such as breast tenderness, nausea, and fatigue, two to three days after you took the second set of pills.

✶ You are still cramping and bleeding moderately four to five days after taking the medications.

If any of these occur, you will need follow-up care to check whether the abortion is complete. If the pregnancy did not pass, you may be able to repeat the medications or you may need uterine aspiration.

After a successful medical abortion, nausea, breast tenderness, and other pregnancy symptoms go away within one to three days. The vaginal bleeding will get lighter over several days until it is on-and-off spotting. Cramping eases up after a day or two. Rest and take it easy during that time because the bleeding and cramping can take a lot out of you. Refrain from sex for two weeks while your body is healing. Remember, to prevent infection, keep everything out of your vagina for two weeks after. This includes tampons, fingers, and penises. As the bleeding lightens and the pregnancy hormones work their way out of your system, you will start feeling better. By two weeks after an abortion, most women feel fully recovered and return to all their activities, including sex.

Four weeks after the medical abortion, take a pregnancy test. If you take one sooner, it will still be positive because pregnancy hormones hang around in your body for quite some time. To avoid scaring yourself, wait the full four weeks to take one! At that time, all the pregnancy hormones should be gone from your system, and your pregnancy test will be negative.

As of this book's printing, in the following states you can obtain a medical abortion through in-person clinics: Washington State, Oregon, California, Nevada, New Mexico, Minnesota, New York, Vermont, Maine, Colorado, Illinois, Virginia, Connecticut, Delaware, New Hampshire, Rhode Island, New Jersey, Maryland, Massachusetts, Michigan, Hawaii, Wisconsin, Ohio, or Alaska. In these states you can also have virtual care, with the pills shipped discreetly to your address from the following online services:

* heyjane.com
* ineedana.com
* carafem.org

If you do not live in one of the states listed above, use abortionfinder.org to find your closest available providers and online options.

If you cannot find a provider within a reachable distance to you, the following resources can help you:

* aidaccess.org: prescribes and ships abortion pills to all 50 states from outside the United States.
* plancpills.org: resources for providers and online services that ship pills.

If you are doing a self-managed medical abortion and need medical advice or counseling, call the Miscarriage + Abortion hotline, 1-833-246-2632, or go to their website, mahotline.org. Pro-choice clinicians are available there to advise you by phone.

Post-Abortion Care

It is normal to have the blues and feel difficult emotions, including sadness, grief, and depression, after an abortion. While your body recovers in a couple of weeks or less, your emotions can take longer. In the first couple of weeks, the rapid drop in hormones when going from pregnant to nonpregnant is dramatic yet invisible. It is similar to the postpartum blues, but it is also something you may be hiding or keeping secret. Many people in your life probably did not even know you were pregnant to begin with. Be gentle with yourself! What can you do to be kind and loving to *yourself*? How about ice cream, a spa day, calling in sick to work so you can rest? What can you ask of a trusted friend? Caring for yourself in this way will help your recovery be smoother.

If your depression and sadness linger past the first couple of weeks, you can use a post-abortion phone counseling service to support your recovery. The following services are free and have trained, compassionate volunteers answering calls and texts:

* Exhale Pro-Voice: call or text 617-749-2948 from 3–9 PM PST weekdays, 1–9 PM Saturday, or 3–7 PM Sunday. Visit

exhaleprovoice.org for more post-abortion care and self-care information.

* All-Options Talkline: 1-888-493-0092
* Connect & Breathe: 1-866-647-1764

Putting It All Together:
Your Plans A, B, and C

This book has covered your menstrual cycle, birth control options (both hormonal and nonhormonal), STIs and safe sex, vaginal health, female sexual pleasure, consent and boundaries, and pregnancy options. The point of sharing all this with you is that now you have the information you need to make a plan for *you*. If you are going to have or are having penis-in-vagina sex, you need to take care of yourself. You are at risk of pregnancy. If you don't intend to get pregnant right now, *what are you going to do*?

Your plan should have three parts, A, B, and C.

Plan A—Contraception: A deliberate method or technique used to prevent pregnancy. This is your first-line plan to prevent pregnancy.

Plan B—Emergency Contraceptive Pill: If there is contraception failure, such as the condom broke or he took it off midway through sex, or there were missed pills or forgotten patches, this is your second line to prevent pregnancy. It is best to keep these on hand or know how to obtain one when needed, either through a drugstore, pharmacy, or clinic.

Plan C: If you get pregnant, carefully consider your options and the resources available to you, and *choose* what to do.

13

Our Choices

Women's Unplanned Pregnancy Stories

t is hard to imagine what these pregnancy options might really be like and how your decision might impact your life, both in the present and in the years to come. I have collected stories from women who had unexpected pregnancies in their teens or early 20s. One lived in Canada, and the rest were from areas across the United States. In this chapter, these women share about the decision they made, how it went for them, and what happened afterward. These women are all between 30 and 50 years old as I write this, and they speak to how the unplanned pregnancy shaped their lives in the years that followed.

I have included three stories from women who chose each of the three different options. These stories do not encompass the vast range of experiences women may have when raising a child as a young mother, placing a baby for adoption, or having an abortion. But they provide a glimpse into these people's particular experiences and give you a sense of what each option might mean in a real-life way.

Choice #1

Continuing the Pregnancy, Having the Baby, Raising the Child

This is Janie, now 50. Janie was raised in a very religious home and was given no sex education. When she got pregnant at 18, she did what her mother told her to do: left college, got married, and had the baby. Her early years of motherhood were difficult, but as she got older she gained agency over her life, family, and choices.

Please briefly describe the situation around the pregnancy.

It was the summer I turned 18 years old, and I was en route home to Hawaii from my second year of college on the East Coast. I had an extended layover in California to visit relatives and had planned to see a boyfriend I had broken up with the previous year. We were technically broken up but we reconnected.

Come July, I didn't get my period and I started to get nervous. I lived on a small Hawaiian island in a very religious family and couldn't buy a pregnancy test. What if someone saw me? Actually, someone would for sure see me, and the whole island would know. It was not an option.

Once early August came and I headed back to college, I planned another layover with my relatives in California. When I saw my ex, I requested that he get a pregnancy test so I could make sure I wasn't pregnant before I returned to school.

The pregnancy test came back positive and my world spun out of control.

He was thrilled and I was devastated.

I couldn't eat or drink for days. I had no idea how I would tell my parents. I was raised a very strict Christian. I was home-schooled (thus no sex education whatsoever). I was attending a private Christian college on academic scholarship.

This boyfriend had been my first kiss, my first boyfriend, and my first everything. He was eight years older than me, and I was 16 when I met him. Growing up, I had never been taught anything about birth control. I honestly had no education on the topic, and since my friends were all very religious too, there was no sharing of such information. I was miserable. I had loved college. I was considering a degree in speech therapy or biology, with a desire to do medical school. I absolutely thrived being in college. I had As in all my classes. I worked hard and loved to learn. I made many friends and was devastated at the thought of not seeing any of them again.

How did you make your decision?

I thought long and hard about my options. Abortion was completely out of the question. I was raised extremist antiabortion. My family would travel to Washington, DC, every January to participate in the annual anti-*Roe v. Wade* protests at the Capitol. I personally, as a child, had been chained to many abortion clinic entrances. I had been "arrested" multiple times and still have a photo of myself from the front page of the *Boston Herald*, being hoisted on my side by five officers and carried into a paddy wagon at 10 years old.

Abortion was not an option, but I thought I could adopt my baby out. I already knew the baby's father was not the right choice for me and I had a lot of growing up to do. I had big educational dreams and honestly had never been one who wanted to have kids. I didn't doubt I might at some point have children, but it wasn't even on my checklist.

I had an aunt and uncle who had never been able to have kids. They were fun and loving, and I realized what a perfect opportunity this could be. I was excited about the option. I discussed the idea with my mom on the phone, and she quickly shot it down. She said I had created this situation and I needed to follow through in the responsible way. I needed to marry the baby's dad. I was heartbroken but I didn't even think twice about the plan she dictated.

We got married in October. I was five months pregnant but, lucky for my mom, not showing at all.

I tried to make the best of my situation. I knew almost no one in California and was embarrassed to stay in contact with my religious friends in college. I looked into classes at the local community college. I was able to enroll in an immunology class at Stanford and loved it. It was the highlight of my week.

The baby was born in March, and from then on I was a mama. I put on a good face and moved ahead with all the courage I could muster. I knew I would make the best of it and everything would be okay. I was a good mom. I ended up getting into a counselor at around 20 years of age. I had just decided I needed to leave my husband. He was controlling and getting more erratic. I started to quietly make plans to leave him, and then I discovered I was pregnant again. That was my second daughter, and I left my husband soon after her birth.

After years as a single mother of two daughters, I had a long-term boyfriend. I was worried about getting pregnant, so when he offered to get a vasectomy, I jumped on it. He had the procedure done and I was thrilled. But the vasectomy failed, and a few months later, I was pregnant. I had an abortion. My daughters were around 12 and 15 then. That boyfriend did not want kids and gave me the support I needed. I had recently completed my bachelor's degree and was getting a master's. I had been in therapy for many years and grown into myself.

I was able to make an informed decision that I've never regretted since.

I went to Planned Parenthood (which I had picketed as a child for years), took the pills, and all went smoothly. I was curious to see if I would have gnarly regret and guilt and pain like I had always been taught abortions caused. I was prepared for it but still knew I did not want another kid.

Shockingly, I felt fine post-abortion.

I didn't have guilt or pain or any of the negative aftermath I was taught.

Looking back from your current age, how did the pregnancy impact the longer trajectory of your life?

Both of my daughters are fully grown and wonderful. I adore them and am so grateful I have them. I worked very hard to raise them well—mostly as a single mom. I saved to get them through college, and they have both graduated with degrees. There were years of pain and grief, but now I am a free woman and traveling the world. I own my own business. I've bought my own home and, after many years of being on my own, I have finally met a wonderful man worthy of my energy and adding to my vitality.

My older daughter just had her first baby, and I am over the moon. It was so fun to watch her and her husband anticipate this baby. Her husband was so incredibly supportive and present, it still brings tears to my eyes. To see a conception and birth so wanted and celebrated—made my heart happy. From day one I talked to my girls about sex and options, and they used to laugh at me and say, "Enough, Mom." But I wanted things to be different for them.

If you could go back in time and talk to that young, newly pregnant *you*, what would you tell her?

Honestly, I have no regrets today. Thirty years later and now my girls are grown and on their own. I am established in my life and know what I want and who I am. I live every day to the fullest and I don't take anything for granted. I know my life could have been very different and I don't even know what it would have looked like, but in the end it is my life and it has worked out.

My older self would say, seek out resources and trust that, in the end, life always works out. Do the best you can. When it's your darkest moment, know there will somehow be light at the end of the tunnel. Stay tough, work hard, be kind, and do the best you can.

Fiona, now 52, became a mother at 19. As a queer person, she did not think that having a child would necessarily happen for her. So when she got pregnant, she saw it as an opportunity. This is her story.

Please briefly describe the situation around the pregnancy.

I left high school early and became a world-traveling back-packer, making my way through Asia for a couple of years by myself. I was living in Europe when I got pregnant, traveling with my girlfriend and my boyfriend. We were countercultural, bisexual, and broke. A woman I'd had a crush on back in California had been a young mom, and I used to babysit her son and carry him around on my hip, pretending I was his mother. Abortion had been legal my whole life and I was pro-choice, but I always hoped I'd be a young mom.

How did you make your decision?

When I realized I was pregnant I didn't give abortion much thought. I was pro-choice, but I wanted to be a mother. I think I knew by then that I was more gay than bisexual, and in those days I didn't know any queer people with kids. So I think I saw this unexpected pregnancy as my opportunity to become a mother.

Did you feel supported by your health care team or by others?

Well, I didn't have a health care team. I was traveling and uninsured. When I finally got in for some medical care, I was in Italy. They called me a gypsy, and not in the proud heritage kind of way. The doctors and nurses mostly mocked me or seemed vaguely horrified. I turned 19 shortly after I got pregnant, and I think if I'd been married and not been countercultural or, you know, owned shoes, they would have been a little bit more respectful. But I was the crazy barefoot American.

How did becoming a mother impact the following three to five years of your life?

I'd hoped to just put the baby on my back and keep traveling, à la Margaret Mead. But my girlfriend had left, my boyfriend's alcoholism was getting out of control, and basically I was just

getting tired. I decided to go back to California to be near my
parents and go back to school. I figured I could balance child-
rearing and college while my daughter was a preschooler, and
that honestly worked out quite well.

Poverty was a problem, but I already knew how to find
free food. Worries about not being able to pay the rent kept
me up at night. My mother really vacillated between being
sort of helpful—babysitting and whatnot—and just being
really shamed and weird about the whole thing. I think my
mother worried it made me look stupid, like I didn't know
how to use birth control. I saw myself as a bohemian. Maya
Angelou had been a teen mom. I made a practice of challenging people's attitudes.

It was such an unquestioned belief in the United States that
teen motherhood was bad, that nothing good could come of
it. Feminists thought I was wasting my life and Republicans
thought I was threatening their way of life somehow. To say
anything positive about teen motherhood was seen as "encour-
aging" it. So ridiculous.

Obviously no one should become a mother against her will,
but what would happen if we just supported each other? I had
my first child when it was best for my physical health but not
the best financially.

How did it impact the longer trajectory of your life?

Being a young mother really focused me. While most of my
peers spent their 20s partying to the edge of their own good
health, I finished college and grad school and had a career by
the time I was in my late 20s. I did have another child 17 years
later with a sperm donor, and in some ways being an older mom
is easier, but the ease is largely because I don't have to deal with
the social meanness. People used to call CPS on me for no rea-

son. Nobody has ever called CPS on me as an older mom, and believe me, kid #2 was mud covered more often than kid #1.

If you could go back in time and talk to that young, newly pregnant *you,* what would you tell her?

It's going to be fine. Stay true to you. College is a good idea. Single motherhood is better than a partner who makes you feel like shit. Stay focused. And if anyone tells you that you can't do whatever you want to do, say, "Just watch me." *Let the rebellion of youth become your superpower.*

Elizabeth, now 37, found herself with an unintended pregnancy at 22. She already had an 18-month-old baby and was struggling in her relationship with her boyfriend. This is her story.

Please briefly describe the situation around the pregnancy.

When I became pregnant with my second child, I was 22 years old and had an 18-month-old baby. We were very poor at the time but were lucky enough to have a house to live in that was provided by my grandparents. My relationship with my partner was on the rocks. He didn't work, played video games all day, was emotionally volatile, and was an alcoholic. I had just gotten a job working at an after-school program, which really saved us financially even though it was a meager paycheck.

How did you make your decision?

I absolutely considered all my options when I got that positive test. I remember just sobbing and sobbing because I didn't feel ready to do it all over again, especially with my relationship in such a bad place. We didn't have much support from family, and I felt very alone. I ultimately decided to proceed with the pregnancy because I had confidence in myself as a mother, and even though he wasn't a great partner for me, my boyfriend really loved our son. He assured me that even though our relationship was rocky, we could make it work.

How was your experience of the pregnancy and birth?
The birth of my second child will always stand out as the most empowering moment of my life. He was born at home, into my own hands, in the water. My birth team provided me with great care, and even though he was the biggest of my babies, he was the easiest to birth! My postpartum healing went very smoothly and I adjusted well to having two little ones. I rode the high of my triumphant birth for quite some time—perhaps I still do!

How did it impact the following three to five years? And beyond that?
Even though the birth and postpartum went so well, things with my partner came to an end when our new baby was about two years old. It was as if the pregnancy and birth bought us a few more years together. We would have separated earlier if I hadn't gotten pregnant again.

Looking back now, I can see that a lot of my own needs and goals were put on hold. It took me about 10 years to get through community college and get my associate's degree. I was and am a fully devoted mother, and my identity is firmly anchored in motherhood, which I love! I can see now that I learned a lot from my kids and in so many ways we have grown up together. I do wish that their early life hadn't been so turbulent, but I can only imagine it would have been a lot worse if I hadn't taken the leap to separate from their dad. He is now sober and happily remarried with stepkids and a new baby. I also remarried 10 years later and then had my daughter. We have a good relationship now and get our families together for dinners and support each other quite a bit.

If you could go back in time and talk to that young, newly pregnant *you,* what would you tell her?
I would tell her to trust her intuition, reach out for help, utilize the community resources, and find a good therapist. I'm actually really proud of how I navigated some very challenging situations and grew into a strong, healthy woman.

Choice #2

Continuing the Pregnancy and Placing the Baby for Adoption

Selah, now 35, got pregnant at 16. She placed her baby for adoption, and this is her story.

Please briefly describe the situation around the pregnancy.

I had just celebrated my 16th birthday when I found out that I was pregnant. I was still in high school, enjoying the growing freedom and being goofy with friends. I was in an off-and-on-again relationship for 10 months prior, but when I found out that I was pregnant it ended our relationship for good. He suggested I choose abortion or adoption because we weren't ready to be parents, and he left. I felt angry and devastated that just months before, he said he would always be there for me, but when I truly needed him, he wasn't.

How did you make your decision to place the baby for adoption? Who gave you support or advice? Did you meet with opposition?

I made my decision to place my daughter in an open adoption plan because I felt like it would give me a chance to grow up myself while providing her with the stable life I wished I had had. I grew up in a home with a struggling single mom. With open adoption I could still be a part of her life. It was a middle ground between closed adoption and parenting. It was a win-win. I would not have chosen adoption without it being open so that I could know how she was doing and so that I could be there to answer her questions as she grew.

I didn't meet any opposition; my family always encouraged me to make an informed decision. I was able to do that by talking to my counselor and finding other teen moms, birth moms, and adoptive parents to talk to. Those conversations opened my eyes to what was possible within adoption and the challenges of teen parenting I hadn't considered.

Her birth father was only involved to sign his rights away. That's the only area I did feel alone at times, grappling with the loss of him not being present and feeling like he didn't care about us. However, I felt very supported and loved by my family throughout my pregnancy and postpartum. I'm grateful I didn't feel alone physically or emotionally, as the friendships of birth moms who I met online, who understood my feelings, were so helpful too.

Did you feel supported by your health care team or by others?

I felt very supported by my health care team, my social worker, my family, and my community. Even teachers showed up for me. I felt respected and advocated for during all my prenatal visits, and during the hospital stay, by everyone I interacted with. We had a birthing plan surrounding my adoption, including holding her and feeding her bottles as much as I wanted, and everyone honored my wishes. I treasured my time with her, knowing these were my days before they would have her for the rest of her life. I took tons of pictures and videos to reflect back on. That time helped me to not have any regrets or feel like I wasted the time I had with her.

My hospital stay is one I look back fondly on, actually, because I felt so surrounded by love and care. I had everyone there who I loved, including both of my parents and my daughter's adoptive parents, whom I had grown to love in the two months of meeting them. It felt like a big family reunion, it felt whole, and I grieved when it was over and we all went our separate ways again.

One of my favorite memories was right before I was about to sign relinquishment papers, when her adoptive parents wanted to talk with me alone. They said, "This is your baby, your decision. We want to make sure that this is really what you want to do. We will be okay if adoption isn't what you feel is best." Giving me that out and permission to change my mind really showed me their heart of ethics and love for *me*, regardless of my baby, and their desire to be parents. For me, this only solidified my choice of *them* as the family I wanted my baby to be raised by.

After placement, I felt a mix of emotions. The biggest one was peace—my heart felt so at peace in the family I had chosen and the open adoption we had decided on together. I was sure of my decision. Yet that didn't stop the grief, the heartache, or the tears. I loved my baby deeply; however, I was sacrificing to give her more than I could at that time in life. It took time to grieve and to work through the grief with counseling and other birth mothers' support, but I have never regretted my decision. I felt gratitude as well for how my story was shaping up, how incredible her parents were, and I had hope for what our future would look like together.

How did this pregnancy impact the following three to five years of your life?

My daughter and her adoptive family were a positive force in my life. I wanted to stay healthy, heal, and move forward in life to make them proud. I was able to finish the goals I had set, including completing high school and going to college. I visited with them several times a year, and we built a really amazing relationship together! My daughter's adoptive parents were positive role models in my life, and I adored still having a front seat to watch her grow. She knew who I was, and my special role in her life was always honored.

Looking back from your current age, how did it impact or not impact the longer trajectory of your life?

I did get pregnant again in college and chose to parent with my now husband. I think being a birth mother, while I had a lot of support and healing, also left a motherhood-sized hole that I couldn't wait to fill. My counselor warned me that statistically that can be common after placement, and it happened. Still, it all worked out! We both received support from my husband's parents to help get us on our feet while also receiving great financial aid to finish college for free *and* with honors.

I feel like my whole life changed after placing my daughter. While it was devastatingly hard at times, it trajected me onto a good path for my life, a different path. I feel like her pregnancy and adoption saved me in a way; it was a second chance at life. I went on to have more children that I parent now with my husband. I wouldn't have gone to that college had I parented her, and I would have never met him. Now my career is one that is satisfying and fits the passions and talents I discovered while healing after adoption.

If you could go back in time and talk to that young, newly pregnant *you*, what would you tell her?

Just breathe. Take a breath and know it will all work out, even if you don't see or understand all the details now. It will come together day by day. And the relationship you have now with your adult daughter and her family is greater than you can ever imagine. *The best is yet to come.*

This is Kristy's story of placing her baby for adoption at age 19. She is now 46.

Please briefly describe the situation around the pregnancy.

I was 18 when I found out I was pregnant for the first time. I was in my first semester of college and still living at home with my parents.

How did you make your decision?

In the beginning I really didn't know what I was going to do and didn't want to make any rash decisions without considering all my options first. Thankfully, my family and friends were very supportive of whatever decision I chose to make. After a couple of months of really considering my options, I chose to pursue adoption. I was not in a position to provide the kind of life I would want for my child, but I knew there was a family out there who could.

I then began working with a local adoption agency that allowed me to interview prospective adoptive couples so I could find a family who I was completely comfortable placing my child with. I chose my adoptive couple about three to four months into my pregnancy. This allowed us to really get to know each other well, and once my birth daughter was born, I had no doubt they were the right couple and parents for her. Since my adoption was/is an open adoption, I have had ongoing contact with my birth daughter since she was born.

During the pregnancy, people would ask about it and I answered based on the situation. If it was a total stranger, I would just tell them that yes, I'm pregnant, and due at the end of April. With other people who I knew better or felt more comfortable around, I would share that I was planning to place my child for adoption in an open adoption. If I got surprised responses from people or the typical response of "I could never do that," I would say, "Well, I really would love to raise this child as my own, but I know that I'm not in a place to provide for her as I would like and hope to, and I'm confident the family I chose for her is fully prepared to do that for her."

How was your experience with giving birth and placing the baby for adoption?

Thankfully I had a wonderful support team during my labor and delivery. My midwife and the hospital nurses were amazing and supported me through the whole process. I was the first one to hold my birth daughter when she was born, and then, when I felt ready, I handed her to her adoptive mom. I spent two days in the hospital, and my birth daughter stayed in my room with me that whole time. I was so thankful for that time I spent with her before she went home with her parents.

How did that decision/event impact the following three to five years of your life?

I was in college when I was pregnant. She was born a week before finals. I took the rest of the week off, the week she was born, and then went back the following week to take my finals. I stayed in college for a couple more years after that.

How did it impact the longer trajectory of your life?

Placing a child for adoption is life-changing! It was and still is the hardest and best decision I have ever made. Once I finally was in a position to start my own family, I was in a good place to become a mother and provide for my children in the way I had always hoped I could. I now have two daughters who I am raising, and all three of my girls have had continuous contact with each other.

If you could go back in time and talk to that young, newly pregnant *you*, what would you tell her?

Finding your support network is truly lifesaving! I was incredibly thankful that I had that. At times the process was incredibly stressful, so maybe knowing everything would really work out for the best in the end would have been amazing!

This is Colette, now 38. She placed a baby for adoption at 25.

Please briefly describe the situation around the pregnancy.

I was 25 years old and a student in university, finishing education to be a teacher, living on a student loan income. I was in Canada in a different province than my parents/family. The birth father and I were close friends "with benefits." We had no intention of being a couple.

How did you make your decision? Did you experience any opposition to your choice?

I made my decision by working with an excellent social worker at Catholic Social Services who shared all my options (raising my baby as a single parent, gifting [placing] my baby, ending the pregnancy) and helped me make an informed decision. Ending the pregnancy was not something I could have personally done. I knew the other two options were both hard. One wasn't harder than the other; they were just different. My social worker encouraged me to "sit on the fence" and wait for the decision to come—feeling each emotion and situation and which one made me feel peaceful.

I decided to gift my baby early in the pregnancy (three months along). I have a strong belief that being a single parent is the hardest job in the world, and most people don't get to choose—it is something that happens to them. I didn't want to be a single parent, and I had the chance to choose.

For the most part, friends and family were very supportive, but I did have some opposition. One person shared that they thought I wasn't taking responsibility for my choices. The two people I thought would be opposed, my two grandmothers, were immediately supportive. I was alone (I was in a different province than my parents) but not lonely. I was in this with the baby, and I felt like we were doing it together. The birth father was supportive and present but didn't come to appointments. He did look at my top three family portfolios, and we picked the same family.

I met the adoptive parents when I was four months pregnant, so most of the pregnancy felt like it was a surrogate pregnancy. It really was a "meant to be" meeting—I felt comfortable with them immediately. The reasons I chose the adoptive couple: They already had a three-year-old son through open adoption and were still in touch with his birth mother, so I figured they would be true to their connection with me; they were both Catholic (like I was), so they both came from big extended families; they didn't live in the same city as I did, so I wouldn't bump into them unexpectedly; they were both teachers; and when I met them I liked them as people.

I appreciated the honesty from the two "parties" that mat-

tered most to me: the birth father and my parents. The birth
father shared the same feelings as me about being in a relationship—we didn't want it and knew we were better as friends. My
parents shared that they would support me however they could
but didn't want to raise the baby if I moved home.

How was your experience of the birth, placement of the child, and recovery?

My social worker was the BEST support ever, making sure I
knew what was coming so that I could be prepared for the emotions that might "hit" me. My doula (labor support) supported
me like an angel (pro bono too). When I was in the hospital after
having the baby and told my doctor that I wasn't ready to leave
on the second day, he fought to let me stay an extra day, even
though the nurses on the floor gave him a hard time.

The birth itself was fast, surreal, and peaceful. A placement ceremony with my parents, the adoptive couple, and a
priest was very spiritual and moving, and it provided a great
passage for me. Even so, leaving the hospital without the baby
was probably the bluest/saddest I have ever felt, but I knew I
was being "carried" by my people and my God. Ten days after,
I called the adoptive parents on the phone to see how things
were going, and it spooked them because in Alberta there is
a 10-day grace period after signing the papers to change your
mind. I called them on the evening of the ninth day without
even realizing it.

Afterward, I recovered at home with my parents for three
or four weeks and remember reveling in the beauty of all of it.
Emotions I experienced were pride, joy, peace, awe, purposeful,
valued, worried, certain, detached, grateful, faithful, vulnerable, and redeemed. Our two dogs (Buster and Truman) were

very therapeutic for me at the time. My social worker prepared me for all the emotions I would feel after childbirth and being in the hospital with a gorgeous newborn. She said I may want to change my mind, but I should only change my decision if serious facts had changed. She didn't want me to change my mind based on these passing emotions.

I went right back to university to finish my degree—it gave me something to focus on right away. I never experienced any ounce of regret at all.

How did that decision/event impact the following three to five years of your life?

I was able to finish my degree and start teaching. It was so exciting to have visits—we had agreed to a couple of visits a year plus e-mails. During our visits I got to love on this little angel— it was a very special and unique situation. I received many confirmations again about my choice/decision—it was right in so many ways. I was able to share my story with people and make them see the beauty of adoption. It helped me be proud and joyful about my decision. It also impacted my faith in a tremendous way.

Looking back from your current age, how did it impact or not impact the longer trajectory of your life?

Placing my child for adoption allowed me to make sure she got the life she deserved, the one I wanted her to have. And I was able to continue with mine knowing she had a beautiful life like I had. I was also proud of the gift I was able to give the adoptive parents—she truly completed their family. I knew God had plans for a family for me—He was going to grant me the desires of my heart, and He did!! I met a wonderful man who adores her and she adores him, and my son and my birth daughter are really close even though they are 10 years apart.

If you could go back in time and talk to that young, newly pregnant *you*, what would you tell her?

Listen to your heart. You got this! Choose joy! My spiritual mentor advised me to be thoughtful about who you share with and choose joy. And I have.

Ending the Pregnancy by Having an Abortion

Grace, now 46, got pregnant at 21. She chose to have a surgical abortion, and this is her story.

Please briefly describe the situation around the pregnancy.

It was about two months before my 21st birthday when I got pregnant. I had been dating my partner at the time for six months, and we were pretty serious. Neither of us enjoyed condoms and I wasn't on the pill, so we were relying on the pull-out method. He was a struggling artist/ex-heroin addict who was 26 at the time, and I was working at a pizza place making close to minimum wage. Not exactly the partnership that lends itself to a viable family dynamic.

How did you make your decision?

When I returned from the clinic with the information that I was pregnant, I resolved to keep the baby and build my life in a way that I never anticipated. I kept thinking how difficult it was going to be. It all seemed like a strange dream, and I was just doing my best to cope with it.

When I woke up the next morning, my stomach sank as I processed the stark reality of what was happening. And then in that moment, I realized that I had another option. I could terminate the pregnancy. I immediately felt lighter and relieved. I told my boyfriend how I was feeling, and he agreed that it was the best thing for both of us. The resolution that I felt that morning never wavered. There was no doubt in my mind that it was the right path for me to take.

How was your experience of the procedure itself?

The procedure was only slightly painful, nothing too terribly bad. My partner came with me and held my hand the whole time. One thing I remember more than anything else was that he wouldn't look me in the eye. I finally said to him "I need you to look at me right now—we are in this together." He was actually really good throughout the whole process. After the procedure I was escorted into the recovery room and given a large pad to wear to monitor my blood loss. When, after about 30 minutes I had no blood to report, they released me and we went home. I had no pain. I was tired but relieved. I never once had second thoughts that this was the right decision for me.

How did the abortion impact the trajectory of your life?

I have absolutely no regrets. Looking back from where I am now at 46, perimenopausal with no desire to ever have children, I am only more and more thankful that I made the decision to terminate my pregnancy. I never have been pregnant again. The thought of having raised a child at that young age and all the ways that my life would be different makes me so grateful for the choice I made. I can't imagine that I ever would've been able to go to Europe or any of the other travel adventures I had in my 20s and 30s. I doubt that I would've gone on to college and gotten my master's degree if I had a teenage kid to worry about. The life that I've lived in the last 25 years would've been wildly different if I hadn't opted to terminate that pregnancy, and I'm so pleased with the child-free life that I have had.

If you could go back in time and talk to that young, newly pregnant *you*, what would you tell her?

Don't waste your time feeling any guilt or shame around this because it's okay. Thankfully you can move past this moment in time and continue to nurture the life you're building. Don't be afraid of the physical pain that you might experience because it's temporary. Use those moments to embrace your realness and your aliveness. Let this be a valuable lesson to make more of an effort to be cautious during sex so that you don't have to be in this position again.

You are strong and powerful, and if/when you decide that you are ready for a child, you can have that. And you will be awesome at it! And if you decide that you don't ever want to have kids, then you'll be even more glad that you didn't go against your instincts to terminate at this time. You've got an amazing, rich, and full life ahead of you—and *YOU are the only being that you should be responsible for right now, so take good care of yourself and keep listening to those instincts. The best relationship you can have is with yourself.*

Rebecca, now 47, had two abortions, one surgical and one medical. This is her story.

Please briefly describe the situation around the pregnancy.

I was 22 years old and I'd been dating the love of my life for less than a year. I knew at the time that we would probably get married someday, but we were so young at the time. Today, 24 years later, we are happily married with two planned children. But at the time, at that young age and so early in our relationship, I'm quite confident that carrying that pregnancy to term would have been the end of our love. The only thing I wanted in life more than motherhood was the freedom to choose when I was ready for it.

At the time I was pretty poor. I was a full-time college student with a part-time job. I had no resources for luxuries or medical expenses, much less raising a child. The cost of the abortion was a stretch, and thankfully I had help.

How did you make your decision?

I suppose there was never any question or doubt about whether I would have an abortion. I certainly wasn't going to have a baby at that point in life. It was unfathomable that I would carry the pregnancy to term. It's not what I wanted, it's not what he wanted, although he said he would support me if it's what I wanted. My recollection is that it was a couple/few hundred dollars, which was a LOT of money that I certainly didn't have. My mother helped pay for it. I can't remember if I told any other friends at the time. Thankfully I had enough support from my mom and the boyfriend, so I may have kept it to myself.

How was your experience of the abortion itself?

I didn't even have a car, so the logistics of getting to the clinic was a hardship. I usually rode my bike everywhere, but I didn't think I'd want to ride a bike home after the procedure. I must have taken a public bus or a taxi. I remember feeling scared yet resolute. And I felt a lot of shame and embarrassment. I know better, I scolded myself. I'm an educated woman and I had access to birth control. Why hadn't I been more diligent about prevention?! How could I have let this happen?!

I remember that everyone at the clinic was kind and supportive. There was no blame or shame from the staff, just empathy and compassion. They recognized that I was scared and tried to offer reassurances. The procedure didn't take long. It was a surgical abortion, and I remember it being unpleasant but not excruciating. I remember being afraid that the procedure might cause permanent damage to my uterus so that later in life, when I wanted to be pregnant, I might have complications.

To be honest, I don't remember much about the procedure. I remember lying on my back with my feet in the stirrups, just like any visit to the gynecologist. And I think the nurse held my hand while the doctor did the procedure. Afterward, in the recovery room, I got nauseous and threw up in a trash can. I remember feeling fragile and wounded. I wasn't physically wounded; it was more like an emotional wound. Or maybe it was a self-imposed penance because the deed deserved the weight of gravity, even if physically I was fine.

How did that decision/event impact the following three to five years of your life?

In the subsequent three years I graduated from college and started my career. I truly feel that neither of those would have been possible if I'd been trying to raise a child. Years later, a wanted pregnancy interrupted my grad school studies, and I never managed to get back to finishing that master's degree.

But a year after that first abortion, we found ourselves

pregnant again. I had just been elected to student government
and had one final year before graduation. The boyfriend and I
kept that second mistake to ourselves and never told even our
dearest friends. One accidental pregnancy was bad enough;
those feelings of shame were even greater the second time
around. This time I didn't even tell my mom or ask for financial assistance. In a way, that extra cost burden was a pun-
ishment I felt I deserved. The boyfriend and I split the cost,
but it meant we couldn't afford any recreational expenses for
about six months. No eating out, no going out with friends,
no fun.

It was hard to believe I was actually pregnant again. Having learned a hard lesson the first time around, we'd been
so diligent about birth control! How could this have happened again?! I honestly couldn't believe it. I was in a state
of shock and kept telling myself it couldn't possibly be true.
And yet the blood test at the health clinic confirmed that I
was pregnant.

Instead of a surgical abortion, they offered me the option
of an [at the time] experimental medication abortion, which
meant I took a couple of pills that would cause the fetus
to abort. It was two years before the FDA would approve
the use of mifepristone. (Must have been a clinical trial?)
I remember being told that this new method usually had a
high success rate but that there was still a chance it might
not be effective. I took the pills literally days before leaving
the country for an internship in Central America. (What if
I got there and found I was still pregnant?!) Far from home
in a foreign country with limited Spanish, I spent the next
week convinced I was probably still pregnant, agonizing
about what my options could possibly be there. Thankfully,
the pills worked.

Looking back from your current age, how did it impact or not impact the longer trajectory of your life?

Motherhood is something I've always wanted, but I didn't want it forced on me then. Parenting requires many sacrifices, and I wasn't ready to sacrifice my dreams and my career path. Frankly, I wasn't willing to sacrifice the motherhood I had always envisioned—and this wasn't it! Motherhood was something I was planning for my future, with the right partner at the right time in my adulthood. I couldn't possibly embark on motherhood while I was still just a child myself!

I suppose it comes from a place of privilege that I should even expect to have choice in such things. It wasn't the privilege of financial wealth but one of expecting to have choices in life. I grew up with the expectation that my path through life would be filled with choices—that I would choose whom to marry and when; that I would have a choice of colleges, choice of studies, choice of career. And a choice about whether and when to become a parent.

As fate would have it, I did end up marrying that same boyfriend. Twenty-four years later, we're still happily married, raising two wanted children. Of course I do think about the babies we could have had back then. Would they be like the two daughters we now have and love? But I never for a minute regret the decision we made at the time to terminate the pregnancies. Parenting is really hard. At least when we're going through the challenging parts, I know I chose this life and these children.

If you could go back in time and talk to that young, newly pregnant *you,* what would you tell her?

I would simply be a steady and supportive ally. *I would remind her that so many millions of other women have also gone through this, and although most of us don't share our stories, she is not alone.* Even if it's the obvious choice, it's still not an easy experience. I would reassure her that it's all going to be okay and that the experience will make her stronger.

Astrid, 54, had an abortion at 19. She agonized over what she should do and ultimately felt pressure from family members and even her health care providers to end the pregnancy.

Please briefly describe the situation around the pregnancy.

I met "Brian" just two days after I got to my college, when I was 19. We were living in the dorms, away from home for the first time. We immediately became very close and spent practically every minute together (when we weren't in class). I kept a journal and have a journal entry from November wherein I wrote, "Brian and I make love all the time and we've been bad about protection. I think I was ovulating yesterday—OOPS!"

My period was always *very* regular—every 28 days. So I was really worried when my period didn't come. My breasts were so tender and I just felt really *off*. I made an appointment for a pregnancy test at the student health center for December 6.

How did you make your decision?

"Sweetheart, you're pregnant," the older nurse practitioner said when she stepped in the room. To this day, I can still see her face and hear her voice.

"WHAT?" I replied. I was completely shocked, even though I shouldn't have been. I suddenly grew very cold and began to shake. The room was spinning. She asked if I knew what I wanted to do about the pregnancy.

"I don't know . . ." I replied.

"There *are* options," she said. "You're only 19, in college, with a future ahead of you. I have been pregnant four times, but I only have two children, if you know what I mean."

It took me a minute to realize what she meant.

Brian was waiting outside the health center in the cold, wearing his black leather rocker jacket with his hands in his pockets, looking like a worried and guilty puppy dog.

"I'm five weeks pregnant," I said, falling into his arms and crying.

"Oh my God," he replied, nearly as shocked as I was.

I called my mother as soon as I got back to my dorm room. I grew up in Berkeley, California, and my hippie mother was a "cool mom," the kind you could tell anything. She asked me within the first two minutes of the conversation if I would be getting an abortion in a way that implied *well, of course you're getting an abortion. You're a 19-year-old college student.*

Over the next 10 days or so—until I went home for winter break—I struggled with what to do. I had wanted to be a mom as long as I could remember and had always romanticized being pregnant. I felt so overwhelmed by this gigantic decision that was looming over me; I was so torn. No one could really help. I wanted someone to just *tell* me what to do, but this huge decision was really up to me—no one could make the decision for me. Brian was very passive and just said he would support me in any decision I made. I spoke to my girlfriends about it. I recall sitting on the floor of a new friend's dorm room, talking about the big decision with her and another new friend.

"We think you should keep it," one of them said. "We don't think you could handle an abortion—it's so obvious you want to be a mom."

I was taken aback. *It shows?* I was suddenly terrified of carrying a baby to term and becoming a mother when I was 19.

It felt like one minute I was carefree and on my own for the first time, newly in love and going to college classes, and then—in the next minute—I was forced to make the biggest decision of my life. My world was so heavy and intense. I cried a lot by myself and in Brian's arms.

When I got home for winter break, I visited my dad in San Francisco and spilled the beans. He looked like he had stuck his finger in a light socket, physically jumping when I told him.

"Princess, you *have to* get an abortion," he said, immediately grabbing the big phone book to look through the yellow pages and call for an appointment right then and there.

Dad said he would pay for it. Part of me really *did* want to be able to return back to my college after break without this huge mess on my plate. It seemed like the majority of the votes were to have an abortion, and I kept coming back to it not being the right time to have a baby. I didn't do well in high school and had practically begged the dean at my college to let me in that past spring. We had become first-name basis, and the thought of letting him down in this way just mortified me.

How was your experience of the abortion itself?

My mother suggested a clinic in Oakland because her friend worked there. I found myself making the appointment with my mom standing next to me.

I woke up the morning of my procedure—December 21—crying and throwing up from morning sickness. I didn't want to have the abortion and I did want it—*both*.

The waiting room was crowded full of women of all ages and races waiting for their names to be called, not speaking to one another. Brian and my mom were on either side of me. I was the only one in the waiting room crying. I couldn't stop.

"I will support you and Brian and the baby if you don't

want to do this," my mother suddenly offered. She hadn't said this before. *Why is she saying this now?* I felt so shaky and depleted, I couldn't even try to formulate that into where I was at right then—already at the clinic, about to have the abortion. It had felt so hard to get there, I didn't want to start over with trying to decide. Images of me living back home again at my mom's with a little baby flashed before my mind. I had been so happy to leave home and start on my own that past August.

My mom's friend stood at my side, holding my hand, as I lay on the exam table with my feet in stirrups and a paper drape over my legs and hips. They had asked me if I wanted my mom or Brian to come in, but for some reason I didn't want them to. This facility had told me on the phone that they don't do any kind of sedation. "We show the women breathing techniques; we find that breathing through it really helps the best." I was wishing I had something to knock me out. I was choking and hiccuping from crying so much, I couldn't really focus on the breathing.

I watched the older male doctor put gloves on his hands and then he first went to check the size of my uterus by putting two fingers inside my vagina while he pushed on my lower belly with his other hand. The next thing I knew, the doctor went to inject numbing medicine into my cervix. I instinctively closed my legs, weeping out loud. It really hurt.

"I don't think I can do this one," he said, rolling back toward the wall on his wheeled stool.

This one.

"She'll be OK," my mom's friend—called the "advocate"— reassured the doctor. "Just give her a minute." She then began to lay it on thick with the breathing exercises, getting close to my face.

"I haven't done anything yet to disturb the pregnancy," the doctor apprised in a kind voice. "You don't have to do this if you don't want to."

I'm back to choosing again? I thought. *NOW?*

"I don't know, I don't know," I started repeating, continuing to cry. And then I said, "Just do it."

I felt the cramping as he dilated my cervix. And then the machine came on and it was so, so loud. I pulled my hand away from the advocate and placed my palms on my lower abdomen. I could feel my whole lower pelvis vibrating from the machine. It was much more painful than I had anticipated. I cried out, saying, "Ouch, it hurts."

When it was over, I was brought into a room with a few cots. I felt like I was in shock—floating—and unable to speak. I lay down and curled into the fetal position, and then in walked Brian and my mom. They both put their hands on me, comforting me.

When we got home, Brian and I lay on my bed, with me crying. I felt such a huge, vacant emptiness. *Would I ever be the same again?*

Two or three days after the procedure, I was bleeding heavily and passing large clots. The cramping was so bad. I put a large clot in a jar, and my mother drove me back to the clinic. It was hard to be physically back in that building. A lady took the jar and disappeared behind the STAFF ONLY door.

"It was definitely products of conception," she said maybe 10 minutes later. *Products of conception?* I thought. It took my brain a few minutes to understand what she meant. "Between this and what came out at your procedure, it might be that you had twins." My stomach dropped. The thought that perhaps there were two made it so much worse.

**How did that decision/event impact the following three
to five years of your life?**

I went back to my dorm in January, hoping that being back at
college would make my pain and loss go away. I started drinking a lot, saying to myself that if I were still pregnant, I couldn't
drink and have fun—telling myself that I should feel relieved
and happy about it.

In the months that followed, I had terrible insomnia and
depression. I didn't want to leave my dorm room. I couldn't stop
thinking about how far along I would have been at this time.
Brian was very sweet and supportive. He and I moved into a little one-bedroom apartment at the end of spring semester. By this
time I had it in my head that I *must* get pregnant again. It was
going to be the one and only thing to make the sadness go away.
I told myself I made a terrible mistake by having the abortion.

I found out I was pregnant with our son on August 6 that year,
incidentally the same month that the baby—or babies—from the
first pregnancy would have been born. Brian and I were still
students—and both working at a mom-and-pop burger joint in
town. I was elated. I didn't really completely put it together at
the time that I was getting my do-over; I got to make the choice I
wish I had made on December 21, when the doctor said, "I don't
think I can do this one."

I relished in the pregnancy—even with terrible nausea and
vomiting—loving every minute of it and keeping a prenatal
diary, wherein I wrote about the beautiful little being growing
inside of me. Brian—just 20 years old like me—was very loving and supportive despite being a little shell-shocked. Our son
was born in April, and I absolutely loved (love) him more than
anything in the world. It was a lot to take on so young, both still
college students and working for minimum wage. We went on to

have another boy two years and five months later. Their names start with the same letter, like twins.

Looking back from your current age, how did it impact or not impact the longer trajectory of your life?

Today I am a nurse. Unlike my cohorts who started college that same year that *I* started, it took me quite a while to get my degree. I took college courses here and there when the boys were little and did not return full time until I was 27. I am absolutely pro-choice and always was. Still, not a December 21 goes by without thinking of that day and of what might have been. However, it has always brought me comfort to know that, had I not had the abortion that day, my older son wouldn't be here. He is 33 now and has grown up to be such an amazing man. He has a little girl now and is a wonderful father.

If you could go back in time and talk to that young, newly pregnant *you*, what would you tell her?

Each woman—or young girl—has her own unique experience when confronted with an unplanned pregnancy. There is no right or wrong way to deal with it, and we all do the best we can do to make that big decision—a decision that can be very difficult for one woman while easy and straightforward for another. Even though abortion was very emotionally painful for me, I completely stand behind the woman's right to choose, and I firmly believe that it should be available for *ALL* women and girls who face the upending experience of an unplanned or unintended pregnancy.

It's My Wrap-Up

At the end of the clinic day, the last clients have picked up their emergency contraceptive pills, left urine samples for STI testing, and gotten their Depo-Provera shots. The instruments I used for IUD insertions are in the autoclave, getting sterilized for tomorrow. I confirm that we let the health department know we treated a syphilis case today. As the sunset spills gold and indigo color across the sky, I finish my charting. I drape my lab coat over my chair, power down my humming computer, thank my staff, and walk out into the softening evening light.

In a perfect world, men would take equal responsibility for pregnancies that are the products of their sperm. We don't yet live in that world, and in fact some men discourage women from using birth control and other safe sex measures. So we women and girls must take care of our own bodies, our own selves.

Sex can be a healthy and pleasurable part of our lives when we empower ourselves with knowledge, agency, and good decision-making. We can trust our inner voices, make a plan for contraception we feel good about, and take the steps needed to put that plan in place. We can select sex partners we can communicate our needs to and with whom we feel respected and considered. We can hold boundaries and say no when something doesn't feel right. And when something unexpected or unplanned happens, we can move through self-blame and get the help we need to heal, recover, and move forward with our lives. Dear readers, taking care of ourselves in this way is the meaning of self-love. Your number one love affair is *you with you*, and it is the only relationship you will ever have that is guaranteed to last a lifetime.

Acknowledgments

I cannot change the march of regressive politics that is erod-
ing reproductive rights in the United States right now. "What
can I do?" I asked myself when *Roe v. Wade* was overturned.
My answer is this book. I have poured everything I know about
birth control and reproductive health into these pages in hopes
that the information will be distributed wherever it serves.
This is not the time for reproductive health care providers to
hold our cards close to our chests. I want to thank everyone
who has supported me in my career, my writing, and the leave I
took to write this book.

Thank you—

To my teachers, mentors, and guides who have shaped me
into the nurse-midwife I am today.

To my sister midwives through the years—Sarah, Cynthia,
Ellie, Diane, Paula, Tuesday, Amber, Kavita, Elena, Jessica. I
love you, and I love how we always have each others' backs!

Same with my writing friends: Ariel Gore, the Binders, Kate Evans, my She Writes community, Catherine Newman, Judy Ann Nock, and Annabel Monaghan. Such sisterhood.

To the brave women who shared their stories for this book.

To my clients and their families who have entrusted me with their lives, their care. You have been and will continue to be my greatest teachers.

To my friends who especially supported me in this project: Ali, Diego and Beth, James, and the kind family of Mana Kai Camping, San Ignacio, Belize.

To my friends who always listen and support me: Serra, Kelly, Jacia, Amanda, Theresa, Holly, Nicole, Baba, and Samantha.

To Katrina Cantrell and the amazing folx of Women's Health Specialists, who keep reproductive health care in Northern California accessible through thick and thin. In my tenure with them, that thick and thin included the Trump presidency, our catastrophic Camp Fire of 2018, a global pandemic that shut down the world, and the reversal of *Roe v. Wade*. Thank you, Lorrie, Erin, Chris, Cindy, Molly, Sally, Dr. Marjorie, MariKathryn, Maria, Nel, Lydia, Sherie, Rebekah, Thais, and all the helpers who come through. Deep bow to you, my peeps forever!

To my agent, Laura Yorke, who said yes, it's a great idea.

To the good people of Countryman Press, who said yes, we want this book.

To my amazing family: my siblings Amy and Brian, Grandpa Marvin, Dr. Tiffany, and the little As.

And to the wider family, Dr. Sarah, Nancy and Mark, Josh and Kelly, Carol and Bill.

To my daughters, Clarabel and Sophia, my love for you informs everything I do.

In loving memory of Betty Raskoff Kazmin: mother, wife,

teacher, and lifelong supporter of reproductive rights. She would be so proud.

To all you readers, for learning to respect yourselves and others.

May my words go wherever they are needed!

Index